Evidence-based Care for Breastfeeding Mothers

Mapped to the UNICEF Baby Friendly Learning Outcomes, this new edition of Pollard's essential textbook ensures readers are equipped with the essential knowledge and skills to effectively promote and support breastfeeding mothers.

Breastfeeding is a major public health issue. Not only does breastmilk provide all the nutrients a baby needs for their first six months, but research shows it also helps to protect infants from infection and reduce obesity, as well as helping to protect mothers from some diseases in later life. Although many women want to breastfeed, rates drop rapidly in the first days and weeks after giving birth. Women need the support of their midwives and health visitors when establishing breastfeeding and throughout their children's infancy. This comprehensive and accessible text covers:

- anatomy and physiology;
- building relationships;
- essential skills and good practice guidance;
- dealing with common problems;
- public health considerations;
- mothers needing additional support;
- babies with special needs; and
- complementary feeding and weaning.

Suitable for midwifery and nursing students, as well as practitioners undertaking continuing professional development, *Evidence-based Care for Breastfeeding Mothers* is designed to aid learning. Each chapter begins with specific learning outcomes linked to the Baby Friendly Learning Outcomes, key fact boxes, clinical scenarios and activities.

Maria Pollard is Deputy Director (Nursing, Midwifery and Allied Health Professions) at NHS Education for Scotland, UK.

Evidence-based Care for Breastfeeding Mothers

A Resource for Midwives and
Allied Healthcare Professionals

Third Edition

Maria Pollard

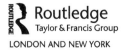

Routledge
Taylor & Francis Group

LONDON AND NEW YORK

Designed cover image: Getty Images

Third edition published 2024
by Routledge
4 Park Square, Milton Park, Abingdon, Oxon, OX14 4RN

and by Routledge
605 Third Avenue, New York, NY 10158

Routledge is an imprint of the Taylor & Francis Group, an informa business

First edition published by Routledge 2011

Second edition published by Routledge 2017

British Library Cataloguing-in-Publication Data
A catalogue record for this book is available from the British Library

ISBN: 978-1-032-25258-2 (hbk)
ISBN: 978-1-032-25240-7 (pbk)
ISBN: 978-1-003-28234-1 (ebk)

DOI: 10.4324/9781003282341

Typeset in Sabon
by Apex CoVantage, LLC

Contents

vi *Contents*

Preface

Healthcare professionals' lack of knowledge and skills to support mothers to breastfeed their infants has been identified as a major contributing factor to low rates of initiation and duration of breastfeeding, leading to inconsistent and inaccurate advice (Renfrew *et al.*, 2005). This is a key public health problem for society and therefore has major implications for service providers, as well as universities, in relation to how students are taught about breastfeeding within the pre-registration curriculum and how midwives, health visitors and other healthcare professionals keep themselves up to date.

Marks and O'Connor (2015) have suggested that midwives are exposed to similar experiences of breastfeeding and cultural influences, as the mothers they care for, which may therefore affect professional practice in both positive and negative ways. There have been a number of studies carried out to identify the reasons for midwives' lack of knowledge and skill, most of which culminates in recommendations being made to improve post-registration education related to breastfeeding (Renfrew *et al.*, 2005; McFadden *et al.*, 2007). However, it was not until the introduction of the UNICEF UK Baby Friendly Initiative (BFI) *Best Practice Standards into Breastfeeding Education for Student Midwives and Health Visitors* (UNICEF UK BFI, 2002, updated 2014) and more recently the *UNICEF UK Baby Friendly Initiative University Standards (2019)* – (see Appendix 1) and the explicit inclusion of breastfeeding in the 2019 *NMC Standards of proficiency for midwives* – (see Appendix 2) that the focus has moved to pre-registration education.

These initiatives have provided guidance and structure for pre-registration curricula and for continuous professional development through a structured accreditation process which includes education of staff.

Renfrew *et al.* recommended that:

> Universities should be fundamental in providing opportunity for pre and post registration education for all health professionals, perhaps adopting the *UNICEF UK Baby Friendly Standards for Pre-registration Education . . .* as a framework, and developing self-study approaches and close links with clinical areas to enable supervised practice.
>
> (2005, p. 87)

In January 2022, 36 per cent of midwifery pre-registration programme and 15 per cent of health visiting programmes had full UNICEF UK Baby Friendly accreditation.

Evidence-based Care for Breastfeeding Mothers: A Resource for Midwives and Allied Healthcare Professionals is based on the UNICEF UK BFI University Standards, which were updated in 2019. The standards continue to build on the 'Ten steps to successful breastfeeding', including a number of changes particularly in relation to building strong mother–baby and family relationships for all. This edition reflects the changes and addresses the following 5 themes and 16 learning outcomes detailed next to ensure that students, midwives, health visitors and other related healthcare professionals are equipped with essential knowledge and skills to enable them to support breastfeeding mothers through the application of evidence-based knowledge to clinical situations.

Theme 1: Understanding breastfeeding

1 Have sufficient knowledge of anatomy of the breast and physiology of lactation to enable them to support mothers to successfully establish and maintain breastfeeding.
2 Understand the importance of human milk and breastfeeding to the health and well-being outcomes of mothers, babies and the wider family.

Theme 2: Support infant feeding

3 Have an understanding of infant feeding culture within the UK and the various influences and constraints which impact on women's infant feeding decisions.
4 Be able to apply their knowledge and understanding of the physiology of lactation to support women to get breastfeeding off to a good start.
5 Be able to apply their knowledge of physiology and the principle of reciprocity to support mothers to keep their babies close and respond to their cues for feeding, love and comfort.
6 Have the knowledge and skills to support mothers and babies to maximise breastmilk and breastfeeding, to continue to breastfeed for as long as they wish and to introduce solid foods at an appropriate time.
7 Be able to support parents who formula feed to do so responsively and as safely as possible.
8 Understand the importance of the WHO International Code of Marketing of Breast-milk Substitutes and subsequent WHA resolutions (the Code) and how it impacts on practice.

Theme 3: Support close and loving relationships

9 Develop an understanding of the importance of secure mother-infant attachment and the impact this has on their health and emotional wellbeing.
10 Be able to apply their knowledge of attachment theory to promote and encourage close and loving relationships between babies, their mothers and families, irrespective of their feeding method.

Theme 4: Manage the challenges

11 Be able to apply their knowledge of the physiology of lactation and infant feeding to support effective management of challenges which may arise at any time during breastfeeding.
12 Have an understanding of the special circumstances which can affect lactation and breastfeeding (e.g. when mother and baby are separated, including preterm and sick infants) and be able to support mothers to overcome the challenges.

13 Draw on their knowledge and understanding of the wider social, cultural and political influences which undermine breastfeeding, to promote, support and protect breastfeeding within their sphere of practice.

Theme 5: Promote positive communication

14 Have an understanding of the principles of effective communication and current thinking around public health promotion strategies and approaches.
15 Be able to apply their knowledge of effective communication to initiate sensitive, compassionate, mother-centred conversations with pregnant women and new mothers.
16 Have the knowledge and skills to access the evidence-based information that underpins infant feeding practice and know how to keep up-to-date (e.g. e-alerts, research summaries).

(Appendix 1 provides a breakdown and further explanation of the components of each outcome.)

The book begins by putting breastfeeding into its socio-political context, leading to a chapter focusing on building relationships and responsive feeding. This chapter is followed by a chapter outlining the essential knowledge and skills required to promote, initiate and support breastfeeding mothers in the early days. This leads on to the management of common problems and supporting breastfeeding mothers and babies with special needs, including alternative methods of infant feeding when breastfeeding is not possible. This is followed by a look at older babies, regarding when and how to commence weaning, and ongoing support of mothers in the community. The book concludes with a chapter on developing knowledge and skills to support breastfeeding mothers using a trauma-informed approach and when required that reasonable adjustments are made to share information in an understandable way for all mothers.

Each chapter is mapped to the appropriate UNICEF UK BFI (2019a) University Standards themes and learning outcomes, and the main text is evidence-based, relating the theory to clinical practice. However, it is evident that in many areas of breastfeeding management, there is still a lack of robust evidence. Each chapter includes key fact boxes, clinical activities, diagrams and photographs when appropriate. Each chapter is consolidated with a quiz, scenarios or reflective questions, and answers to these are found at the end of the book. Useful resources are also listed at the end of each chapter with a complete reference list and a glossary at the end of the book.

I would like to thank the following for giving permission to reproduce material: Medela, Karen McKay NHS Highland, TIPS Lancet Series- Rollins et al, Oot et al and NHS Education for Scotland and special thanks to the UNICEF UK BFI.

A special thank you to Tony, Thomas and Andrew for their encouragement throughout my career and my Mum and Dad for giving me the best start to life.

Maria Pollard

Abbreviations

ABM	Association of Breastfeeding Mothers
AED	anti-epileptic drug
APGAR	appearance, pulse, grimace, activity, respiration (from Apgar, its inventor)
ARV	antiretroviral
BAPM	British Association of Perinatal Medicine
BFI	Baby Friendly Initiative
BFLG	Baby Feeding Law Group
BFM	Breastfeeding Manifesto
BFN	Breastfeeding Network
BMA	Baby Milk Action
BMI	body mass index
BPA	bisphenol-A
DH	Department of Health
FIL	feedback inhibitor of lactation
FSA	Food Standards Agency
FSID	Foundation for the Study of Infant Deaths
GP	general practitioner
HCV	hepatitis C virus
HE	higher education
HEAT	health improvement, efficiency, access, treatment
HPL	human placental lactogen
HSE	Health and Safety Executive
IBFAN	International Baby Food Action Network
IFAS	Infant Feeding Attitude Scale
LAM	lactational amenorrhoea method
NAS	neonatal abstinence syndrome
NCT	National Childbirth Trust
NICE	National Institute for Health and Clinical Excellence
NMC	Nursing and Midwifery Council
PCOS	polycystic ovary syndrome
PIF	prolactin-inhibiting factor
RCM	Royal College of Midwifery
RCOG	Royal College of Obstetricians & Gynaecologists
SACN	Scientific Advisory Committee on Nutrition
SCBU	special care baby unit
SG	Scottish Government

SIDS	sudden infant death syndrome
sIgA	secretory immunoglobin A
SIGN	Scottish Intercollegiate Guidelines Network
SPS	Specialist Pharmacy Service
TAMBA	Twins and Multiple Births Association
TB	tuberculosis
UK	United Kingdom
UKAMB	United Kingdom Association for Milk Banking
UNICEF	United Nations Children's Fund
WABA	World Alliance for Breastfeeding Action
WHA	World Health Assembly
WHO	World Health Organization

1 Putting breastfeeding into context

- Learning outcomes
- The benefits of breastfeeding
- Economic and environmental factors
- Who breastfeeds?
- UNICEF UK Baby Friendly Initiative
- Global and national strategies
- Breastfeeding in public
- Concluding comments
- Practice questions
- Resources

Breastfeeding cannot be considered as a standalone subject when culture, social support and healthcare professionals' knowledge and skills clearly have such a great impact on initiation and duration of breastfeeding rates in the United Kingdom (UK) (Renfrew *et al.*, 2005, 2012; Victora *et al.*, 2016; Rollins *et al.*, 2016; Gavine *et al.*, 2016). Breastfeeding must be placed in the wider socio-political context to understand why mothers make the choices they do with regard to infant feeding and to enable healthcare professionals to adequately support them in practice. The *Lancet* Breastfeeding series (Rollins *et al.*, 2016, p. 492) describes the determinants of breastfeeding, using the conceptual model in Figure 1.1, which affect women's breastfeeding decisions and behaviours. In addition, they highlight that most women are biologically capable of breastfeeding, but breastfeeding practices are affected by historical, socioeconomic, cultural, and individual factors that must be taken into consideration.

The aim of this chapter is to identify the role breastfeeding has in promoting public health and reducing health inequalities for both mother and infant by exploring the health benefits of breastfeeding and the dangers of not doing so. This chapter also introduces some of the main global, national and local strategies to promote, support and protect breastfeeding.

DOI: 10.4324/9781003282341-1

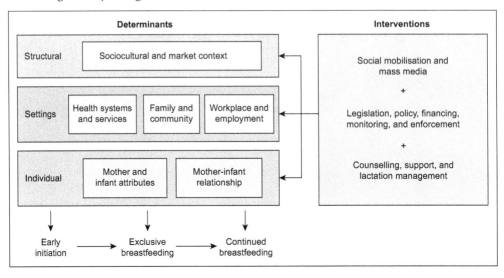

Figure 1.1 The components of an enabling environment for breastfeeding – a conceptual model
Source: Rollins *et al.* (2016, p. 492).

Mapping to UNICEF UK BFI Education learning outcomes (2019a)
   By the end of the programme, students will:

Theme		Learning outcomes
Theme 1: Understand breastfeeding	2.	Understand the importance of human milk and breastfeeding to the health and wellbeing outcomes of mothers, babies and the wider family.
Theme 2: Support infant feeding	3.	Have an understanding of infant feeding culture within the UK and the various influences and constraints which impact on women's infant feeding decisions.
	8.	Understand the importance of the WHO International Code of Marketing of Breastmilk Substitutes and subsequent WHA resolutions (the Code) and how it impacts on practice.
Theme 4: Manage the challenges	13.	Draw on their knowledge and understanding of the wider social, cultural and political influences which undermine breastfeeding, to promote, support and protect breastfeeding within their sphere of practice.
Theme 5: Promote positive communication	14.	Have an understanding of the principles of effective communication and current thinking around public health promotion strategies and approaches.

Learning outcomes

By the end of this chapter, you will be able to:

- identify the health benefits of breastfeeding for mother and infant;
- recognise the socio-economic characteristics of mothers who choose to breastfeed or not;

- describe the BFI best practice standards for healthcare facilities and education; and
- discuss the importance of global, national and local policies and guidelines to encourage and support breastfeeding.

The benefits of breastfeeding

The World Health Organization (WHO, 2021a) recommends exclusive breastfeeding for the first six months of life and to continue for two years and beyond because breastmilk is perfectly balanced to meet the nutritional needs of newborns and is the only food required until six months of age. Breastmilk has the advantage of being readily available, at no cost, and delivered on demand and at the right temperature, and infants are able to regulate the amount required at each feed. The properties of breastmilk are exclusive, cannot be replicated by formula milk (see Chapter 3) and confer many benefits on both mother and infant. Despite this, the WHO (2021a) estimates that only 44 per cent of infants are exclusively breastfed for six months. It is widely accepted that breastfeeding protects against a range of adverse health outcomes (Grummer-Strawn and Rollins, 2015) and supports the mother-baby relationship.

In 2007, Ip *et al.* conducted a systematic review of the evidence on the effects of breastfeeding on short- and long-term infant and maternal health in developed countries. For the infant, they suggested that breastfeeding reduces the risk of diarrhoea and chest infections, atopic dermatitis and asthma, obesity and type I and II diabetes, childhood leukaemia, sudden infant death syndrome (SIDS) and necrotising enterocolitis (NEC).

There have been a number of studies more recently that support Ip's conclusions; the following are a few examples. In a large prospective study of 1,105 children, Silvers *et al.* (2012) found that breastfeeding protected against wheezing in children aged 2–6 years. A meta-analysis carried out by Amitay and Keinan-Boker in 2015 found that any breastfeeding for six months or longer was associated with a lower risk of childhood leukaemia. Colaizy *et al.* (2016) found that if extremely low birth weight infants were not being fed breastmilk, they were at increased risk of NEC.

Kramer *et al.* (2008) suggest a link between intellectual and motor development and 'dose-related' breastfeeding. It is thought this could be due to the long-chain polyunsaturated fatty acids in breastmilk as well as the psychosocial stimulation and bonding conferred by breastfeeding. WHO (Horta and Victora, 2013) commissioned an update of the 2007 systematic review (Horta *et al.*, 2007) of the long-term impact of breastfeeding on health. The evidence from this review could only establish a benefit in the protection against overweight or obesity and an increase in performance in intelligence tests. Evidence was inconclusive on the protection against high total cholesterol and high blood pressure, and conflicting results were found on diabetes.

In 2016, the *Lancet* Series (Victora *et al.*, 2016, and Rollins *et al.*, 2016,.) analysed data from 28 systematic reviews and meta-analyses asserting that the deaths of 823,000 children and 20,000 mothers' breast cancer deaths could be prevented through universal breastfeeding. They indicated that breastfeeding infants for longer periods results in lower infectious morbidity, including diarrhoea and respiratory illness, and mortality, increased protection against child infections and malocclusion, increases in intelligence and probable reductions in overweight and diabetes in later life but it did not find associations with allergic disorders such as asthma, blood pressure or cholesterol (Victora *et al.*, 2016). Rollins *et al.* (2016, p. 1) suggested that 'not breastfeeding is associated with lower intelligence and economic losses of about $302 billion annually or 0·49 per cent of world gross national income'. Furthermore, they state that 'breastfeeding provides short-term and long-term health and economic and environmental advantages to children, women, and society. To realise these gains, political support and financial investment are needed to protect, promote, and support breastfeeding'.

The UK is facing an obesity epidemic that is predicted to increase. The Department of Health and Social Care (DHSC) (2020) state that 63 per cent of adults are above a healthy weight, and of them, half are obese; 1:3 children leaving primary school are overweight, and 1:5 of them are obese. In England between 2006/7 and 2020/21, there has been a disproportionate increase in obesity in children from low-income homes and certain ethnicities (Nuffield Trust, 2022):

- Aged 4–5 years from most deprived (12.2 to 19.7 per cent, respectively) and least deprived (7.7 to 9.1 per cent, respectively).
- Aged 10–11 years from most deprived (21.5 to 32 per cent, respectively) and least deprived (13 to 15 per cent, respectively).

Obesity is associated with an increased risk of hypertension, type II diabetes, heart disease and some cancers. Numerous studies have found that prolonged or dose-related breastfeeding reduces the risk of obesity and that breastfed children are leaner than those who were never breastfed (Yan *et al.*, 2014). The *Childhood Obesity: A Plan for Action* (DHSC, 2016), updated in 2017, states that overweight and obesity-related conditions across the UK cost the NHS £6.1 billion each year with almost 900,000 obesity-related admissions in 2018–19. They suggest a range of initiatives to tackle this crisis, which includes consultation on a proposal to 'help parents of young children to make healthier choices through more honest marketing and labelling of infant foods' but does not include breastfeeding or appropriate weaning.

Breastfeeding also confers benefits on the mother by regulating fertility (Wambach and Riordan, 2016) and reducing the risk of osteoporosis and ovarian and breast cancer in later life, as well as type II diabetes (Ip *et al.*, 2007; Grummer-Strawn and Rollins, 2015). Ip *et al.* (2007) suggest that the protective factors of breastfeeding for mothers are also dose-related; that is, the longer a mother breastfeeds, the better protection she receives, particularly for breast cancer. Victora *et al.* (2016) also found evidence that breastfeeding can prevent breast cancer and improve birth spacing and may reduce the risk of diabetes and ovarian cancer. Ip *et al.* (2007) also suggested that early cessation of breastfeeding or not breastfeeding at all increases the risk of postnatal depression.

In addition, breastfeeding helps mothers return to their pre-pregnancy weight more quickly by utilising the fat laid down in pregnancy for energy. Oxytocin, the hormone involved in the 'let-down' reflex, also causes contraction and involution of the uterus. Breastfeeding immediately following birth assists contraction of the uterus, encouraging placental separation and resulting in a possible reduction in postpartum blood loss (Almutairi, 2021). A small study of 66 mothers in Sweden conducted by Jonas *et al.* (2008) concluded that breastfeeding also reduced both systolic and diastolic maternal blood pressure within two days of giving birth.

Many mothers are now aware that breastfeeding is associated with these benefits. Research continues to identify other diseases that breastfeeding may offer protection against. For example, in a large study of 1 million women, Liu *et al.* (2009) identified that the incidence of gall bladder disease increased by 8 per cent with each birth. However, the risk was reduced by 7 per cent for each year of breastfeeding. Pikwer *et al.* (2008) also suggest that women who breastfed for longer than 13 months were 50 per cent less likely to develop rheumatoid arthritis than those who had never breastfed and 25 per cent less likely if they breastfed for 1–12 months.

Economic and environmental factors

As well as being safe and conferring health benefits, breastfeeding is free and environmentally friendly. A UK All-Party Parliamentary Group (APPG, 2018) inquiry into the financial impact of infant formula milk found that the cost on families was significant. For a 2–3-month-old infant, this ranged from £6.44–£13.52 per week for powdered milk and £24.47–£32.20 per week for ready prepared products. The inquiry collected lived experience evidence from families across the UK in a variety of contexts and reported on the following themes (APPG, p 2):

• The cost of infant formula significantly impacts on some family budgets.
• Families who cannot afford formula may resort to unsafe practices to feed their babies (watering down feeds, adding cereal, early introduction of solids or cow's milk, breast-feeding when contraindicated; see Chapters 7 and 8).
• The small number of families where breastfeeding is contraindicated and who have been advised to formula feed may be at particular risk of hardship.

In 2012, Renfrew *et al.* (2012) were commissioned by UNICEF UK Baby Friendly Initiative (BFI) to undertake an economic analysis of diseases and conditions preventable by breastfeeding. Illnesses that were reviewed included breast cancer in the mother, and gastroenteritis, respiratory infections, middle ear infections and NEC in the baby. They estimated that there could potentially be a saving of £40 million per year: the authors' calculations show that moderate increases in breastfeeding could see millions in potential annual savings to the NHS – and this figure might only be the tip of the iceberg. The report suggested that if half of the mothers who currently do not breastfeed were to do so for up to 18 months over their lives, there would be 865 fewer cases of breast cancer, with cost savings to the NHS of over £21 million. If 45 per cent of babies were exclusively breastfed for four months and if 75 per cent of babies in neonatal units were breastfed at discharge, each year there would be:

• 3,285 fewer babies hospitalised with gastroenteritis and 10,637 fewer general practitioner (GP) consultations, saving in excess of £3.6 million.
• 5,916 fewer babies hospitalised with respiratory illness and 22,248 fewer GP consultations, saving approximately £6.7 million.
• 21,045 fewer GP visits for ear infection, saving approximately £750,000.
• 361 fewer cases of the potentially fatal disease NEC, saving over £6 million.

The key messages arising from the report were:

• Low breastfeeding rates in the UK lead to an increased incidence of illness that has a significant cost to the health service.
• Investment in effective services to increase and sustain breastfeeding rates is likely to provide a return within a few years, possibly as little as one year.

- Investing in supporting women to breastfeed will improve the quality of life for women through the reduction in incidence of breast cancer and for children through reducing acute and chronic diseases.
- Research into the extent of the burden of disease associated with low breastfeeding rates is hampered by data collection methods; this can be addressed by investment in good-quality research.

(Renfrew *et al.*, 2012, p. 7)

Artificial feeding has a larger carbon footprint than breastfeeding. It has significant detrimental effects on the environment and contributes to global warming through cattle grazing and the consumption of fossil fuels in the production, distribution, disposal and waste of formula milk and packaging (WABA, 2005; Linnecar *et al.*, 2014; Palmer, 2017; Karlsson *et al.*, 2019), for example:

- Production of formula milk leads to deforestation of land required to graze cows, which also leads to increased sewage polluting rivers and ground water. Cow flatulence leads to approximately 20 per cent of global methane gas, which contributes to greenhouse gases and global warming.
- Production processes of plastic bottles and teats and other infant feeding equipment leads to increased carbon dioxide emissions and the plastics themselves contain toxins such as bisphenol-A (BPA). It is estimated that they can take up to 450 years to break down in landfill sites.
- Packaging of formula milk involves tins, paper and tetrapaks, most of which is not recycled.
- Transportation of formula milk and feeding equipment to distributors and transportation of purchasers to buy the products use valuable resources.

Because breastfeeding is available at source and on demand, it uses none of the resources listed and therefore does not create any pollution. Furthermore, lactational amenorrhoea in breastfeeding mothers helps reduce family sizes, which improves women's health, while reducing the production, distribution, disposal and waste of products associated with menstruation, such as sanitary towels and tampons.

Oot *et al.* (2021) criticise the United Nations Food Systems Summit 2021 conceptual framework of food systems for diets and nutrition because it does not include breastfeeding as the first human food system. They suggest stakeholders must recognise the barriers to breastfeeding within the food system and that breastfeeding must be recognised as a critical first food (Figure 1.2).

Who breastfeeds?

Statistics provide healthcare professionals with important information about the characteristics of those who choose to breastfeed and for how long. This information enables the development of breastfeeding promotion programmes, policies and guidelines at national and local levels. On an individual level, they also provide healthcare practitioners with an understanding of the reasons women make the choices they do. The last comprehensive UK survey was conducted in 2010. Prior to this, the *Infant Feeding Survey* was conducted every five years to provide estimates on the incidence, prevalence and duration

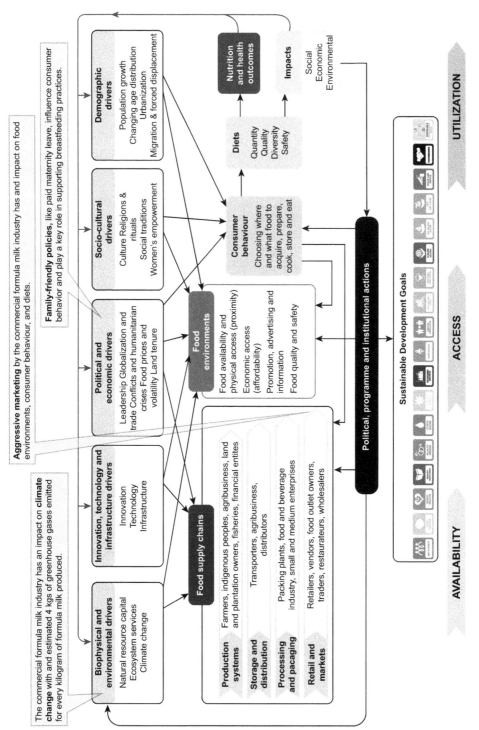

Figure 1.2 How the commercial milk formula industry and regulatory policies influence breastfeeding and the first food system

Source: Oot *et al.* (2021, p. 4).

of breastfeeding; however, the survey was discontinued. Alternative sources of information can be found at:

England	www.england.nhs.uk/statistics/statistical-work-areas/maternity-and-breastfeeding
Northern Ireland	www.niassembly.gov.uk
Scotland	https://publichealthscotland.scot
Wales	https://statswales.gov.wales/Catalogue/Health-and-Social-Care/NHS-Primary-and-Community-Activity/Breastfeeding

In 2017, the Scottish Government (SG) conducted the *Scottish Maternal and Infant Nutrition Survey* to support the implementation of the Maternal and Infant Nutrition Framework for Action (2011), which highlighted an increase in breastfeeding rates at 6 months from 32 per cent in 2010 to 43 per cent in 2017. Similar to *The Infant Feeding Survey 2010* (McAndrew *et al.*, 2012), the *Scottish Maternal and Infant Nutrition Survey* continues to demonstrate evidence of a relationship between breastfeeding and socio-demographic characteristics and the need to focus support in areas of inequalities. There were approximately 2,500 responses at each stage of the survey (antenatal, 8–12 weeks postnatal and 8–12 months postnatal). Although it did not fully replicate the UK Infant Feeding Survey in the question wording, methodology and sampling strategy, it is useful for comparison. It should also be noted that the demographic profile of women giving birth in Scotland has changed since 2010, mothers tend to be older.

The *Scottish Maternal and Infant Nutrition Survey* (SG, 2017) demonstrated

- Three-quarters of respondents to both postnatal surveys had 'ever' breastfed and/or expressed milk for their new baby (75 per cent of the 8–12-week survey and 76 per cent of the 8–12-month survey).
- More than two-thirds of all respondents (69 per cent) were giving breastmilk to their babies when they left the maternity unit.
- Three-quarters of respondents (75 per cent) who had stopped giving breastmilk reported that they would have liked to have given breastmilk for longer. The most reported reasons for stopping breastfeeding or expressing milk were feeding problems (49 per cent), thinking the baby was not getting enough milk (45 per cent) and finding it 'too difficult' (25 per cent).
- Around a quarter of respondents who had stopped breastfeeding or expressing milk thought that access to certain types of support would have helped and encouraged them to breastfeed or express milk for longer.
- 80 per cent of those aged 35 years or older stated that they had intended to give breastmilk (65 per cent breastfeed or express only; 15 per cent mix feed) compared with 57 per cent of 20–24 years (48 per cent breastfeed or express only; 10 per cent mix feed).
- Younger respondents were more likely to have expressed an intention to formula feed only – 35 per cent of respondents aged 20–24 years compared with 15 per cent for those aged 35 years or older.
- Nearly two-thirds of respondents (65 per cent) who lived in the most deprived areas had intended to give breastmilk to their babies compared with nearly 82 per cent of those living in the least deprived areas. More than one in four respondents (28 per cent) who lived in the most deprived areas intended to formula feed compared with just over one in ten (12 per cent) who lived in the least deprived areas.

The common situations that lead to early weaning

Early introduction of solid food increases the risk of ill health for infants and is not recommended until six months of age. Coinciding with changed advice from WHO and the Department of Health regarding the timing of weaning from four to six months of age, the *Infant Feeding Survey 2010* (McAndrew *et al.*, 2012) identified an improvement in the age when parents introduced solid foods into their infants' diet compared with 2005. Nearly seven in ten (69 per cent) of all mothers in the UK introduced solids after four months, and nearly all mothers introduced solids by six months (94 per cent, compared with 98 per cent in 2005) with only 5 per cent of mothers introducing solids after six months (2 per cent in 2005), suggesting mothers were not following guidance on weaning after six months as three-quarters of mothers had already introduced solids by the time their babies were five months old. McAndrew *et al.* (2012) also reported that early weaning was associated with younger age groups of mothers, lower social class groups and lower levels of education. The *Scottish Maternal and Infant Nutrition Survey* (SG, 2017) demonstrated further improvement with 96 per cent of respondents who did not introduce complementary feeding until their infant was at least four months, of whom 46 per cent waited until six months or later. Only 3 per cent of respondents reported introducing solid foods before their babies were four months old compared with 32 per cent in the 2010 survey.

McAndrew *et al.* (2012) reported that overall, the reasons for weaning were similar to those in the 2005 survey (Bolling *et al.*, 2007) in which 52 per cent were broadly influenced by the perception that babies are not satisfied by milk alone (52 per cent). The *Scottish Maternal and Infant Nutrition Survey* (SG, 2017) reported a reduction to 30 per cent who chose this response. Other reasons for introducing complementary feeding before four months and at six months of age or older can be found in Table 1.1:

Table 1.1 Reasons for starting to give complementary foods
(Question asked in survey: Why did you decide to start giving your baby foods other than milk at this age?)

Reason for introducing food other than milk	Age <4 months	Age >6 months
Baby not satisfied with milk	70%	14%
Thought it was the right time	59%	63%
Previous experience with other baby	32%	35%
Baby waking up during the night	26%	7%
Partner/friend/relative advised me	17%	8%
Healthcare professional advised me	14%	59%
Baby able to sit up + hold food in hand	13%	52%
Fun First Foods booklet advised	5%	29%
Read leaflets/info that advised me	2%	41%
Baby not gaining enough weight	1%	2%
Other reason	8%	0

Source: SG (2017, p. 133)

The *Scottish Maternal and Infant Nutrition Survey* (SG, 2017) results are encouraging with a high per centage of respondents taking professional advice and recognising when the infant is ready at six months, but reasons for introducing solid food before four months continue to be of concern. In addition, infant food labels continue to recommend these products as suitable from the age of four months (Crawley and Westland, 2017).

As well as family and friends influencing decisions about weaning, understanding different information about introducing solid food can contribute to early weaning. In England, the Office for Health Improvement and Disparities (OHID, 2022a) commissioned a survey to inform the launch of the Better Health Start for Life Weaning Campaign (DHSC, 2022) and found:

- 40 per cent of parents feel unsure as to what age to start introducing solid foods.
- 41 per cent of first-time mothers introduced solid foods by the time their babies were 5 months old even though experts recommend that solid food should be introduced from the age of 6 months.
- 45 per cent said they found how much food to give their baby confusing.
- 43 per cent found when to progress from certain tastes and textures confusing.
- 64 per cent of parents received conflicting advice on what age to start introducing solid foods.
- 73 per cent agree that there should be one official source for weaning advice.
- 28 per cent of first-time mothers reported that their mother had the biggest influence on their decision to start weaning.

Culture also plays an important role. Some ethnic minority mothers introduce solids by two months of age for similar reasons as stated here but with additional cultural reasons. For example, some mothers thicken breast or formula milk with cornmeal, maize, cereal, rusks or semolina.

Introducing solid food is discussed further in Chapter 10.

UNICEF UK Baby Friendly Initiative

In 1989 the WHO/UNICEF published *Protecting, Promoting and Supporting Breastfeeding: the Special Role of Maternity Services*, which included the *Ten Steps to Successful Breastfeeding* (WHO/UNICEF, 1989) in response to concerns about hospital practices; this was the forerunner to the BFI, 1992. The aim of this initiative was to ensure that pregnant and breastfeeding women had access to high standards of care by supporting healthcare settings to implement best practice standards. In 1998 the *Seven Point Plan for the Protection, Promotion and Support of Breastfeeding in Community Healthcare Settings* was published, reflecting the *Ten Steps*, and was later updated in 2008 and renamed *The Seven Point Plan for Sustaining Breastfeeding in the Community*. In 2017, WHO published *Protecting, Promoting and Supporting Breastfeeding in Facilities Providing Maternity and Newborn Services* as an update to the 1989 document, continuing to build on the guidance of the Innocenti Declaration on the *Protection, Promotion and Support of Breastfeeding* (WHO, 1990) and the Innocenti Declaration 2005 *Infant and Young Child Feeding* and was followed by an update of the *Ten Steps to Successful Breastfeeding* in 2018 (Table 1.2).

Over the years UNICEF UK BFI have updated the Baby Friendly Standards, building on the *Ten Steps to Successful Breastfeeding* and *Seven Point Plan for Sustaining Breastfeeding in the Community*. In 2017 they were further updated in line with emerging evidence to include parent-infant relationships. UNICEF UK BFI provide an accreditation programme for services to demonstrate achievement of the standards to support all mothers with infant feeding. See Table 1.3 or www.unicef.org.uk/babyfriendlyfor further detail.

Table 1.2 The Ten Steps

Ten Steps	
Critical management procedures	
Step 1	a) Comply fully with the International Code of Marketing of Breast-milk Substitutes and relevant World Health Assembly resolutions. b) Have a written breastfeeding policy that is routinely communicated to all healthcare staff. c) Establish ongoing monitoring and data management systems.
Step 2	Ensure all staff sufficient knowledge, competence and skills to support breastfeeding.
Key clinical practices	
Step 3	Discuss the importance and management of breastfeeding with pregnant women and families.
Step 4	Facilitate immediate and uninterrupted skin-to-skin contact and support mothers to initiate breastfeeding as soon as possible after birth.
Step 5	Support mothers to initiate and maintain breastfeeding and manage common difficulties.
Step 6	Do not provide breastfed newborns any food or fluids other than breastmilk, unless medically indicated.
Step 7	Enable mothers and their infants to remain together and to practise rooming-in 24 hours a day.
Step 8	Support mothers to recognise and respond to their infants' cues for feeding.
Step 9	Counsel mothers on the use and risks of feeding bottles, teats and pacifiers.
Step 10	Coordinate discharge so that parents and their infants have timely access to ongoing support and care.

Source: WHO (2018); www.who.int/publications/i/item/9789241550086 (accessed 29 January 2023).

Table 1.3 UNICEF UK Baby Friendly Initiative Standards (2017a)

Building A Firm Foundation	
Stage 1	Have written policies and guidelines to support the standards. Plan an education programme that will allow staff to implement the standards according to their role. Have processes for implementing, auditing and evaluating the standards. Ensure there is no promotion of breastmilk substitutes, bottles, teats or dummies in any part of the facility or by any of the staff.
Stage 2	**An Educated Workforce** Educate staff to implement the standards according to their role and the service provided.
Stage 3	**Parents' Experiences of Maternity Services** Support pregnant women to recognise the importance of breastfeeding and early relationships for the health and wellbeing of their baby. Support all mothers and babies to initiate a close relationship and feeding soon after birth. Enable mothers to get breastfeeding off to a good start. Support mothers to make informed decisions regarding the introduction of food or fluids other than breastmilk. Support parents to have a close and loving relationship with their baby.

(Continued)

Table 1.3 (Continued)

	Parents' Experiences of Neonatal Units Support parents to have a close and loving relationship with their baby. Enable babies to receive breastmilk and to breastfeed when possible. Value parents as partners in care. **Parents' Experiences of Health Visiting Services** Support pregnant women to recognise the importance of breastfeeding and early relationships for the health and wellbeing of the baby. Enable mothers to continue breastfeeding for as long as they wish. Support mothers to make informed decisions regarding the introduction of food or fluids other breastmilk. Support parents to have a close and loving relationship with their baby. **Parents' Experiences of Children's Centres** Support pregnant women to recognise the importance of breastfeeding and early relationships for the health and wellbeing of their baby. Protect and support breastfeeding in all areas of the service. Support parents to have a close and loving relationship with their baby.
Re-accreditation	Embed all the standards to support excellent practice for mothers, babies and their families.

Source: www.unicef.org.uk/babyfriendly

Breastfeeding remains an important part of establishing strong relationships but is not the sole aim of the standards; the focus is on communication styles and a mother-centred approach. Whilst they incorporate the *Ten steps to successful breastfeeding*, there are a number of changes particularly in relation to building strong mother-baby-family relationships for all. Previously debated topics such as *skin-to-skin contact* and *rooming-in* are now part of routine practice, so the new standards reflect a broader approach and respond to the importance of early care practices.

Implementation of the UNICEF UK BFI best practice standards has been identified as a way to increase breastfeeding rates (Entwistle, 2013; Rollins *et al.*, 2016; NICE, 2021a) and has been implemented across the UK. In 2019 Northern Ireland and Scotland had 100 per cent of births in BFI-accredited hospitals followed by Wales at 78 per cent and England at 58 per cent (www.statista.com). Across the UK this equates to 43 per cent of maternity services; 67 per cent of health visiting services and universities, 36 per cent of midwifery courses and 15 per cent health visitor courses (www.unicef.org.uk/babyfriendly, updated January 2022).

Despite the success of these initiatives, concern has been expressed about the level of breastfeeding education for students in pre-registration programmes and why it is necessary for employers to provide additional education for registered midwives and health visitors. This led to the development of the *Best Practice Standards for Higher Education Institutions* in 2002, revised in 2014 and more recently in 2019 (UNICEF UK BFI, 2019a).

The new education standards have five themes and 16 learning outcomes (Table 1.4) to be introduced into the curriculum and successfully achieved at the point of registration as a midwife or health visitor. The intention is to equip students with the tools to be able to communicate successfully with mothers, enable and support parents to make informed choices about infant feeding and build good relationships to give their babies the best start in life.

Table 1.4 UNICEF UK BFI University learning outcomes (2019a) (further details can be found in Appendix 1)

Theme		Learning outcomes
By the end of the programme, students will:		
Theme 1: Understanding breastfeeding	1.	Have sufficient knowledge of anatomy of the breast and physiology of lactation to enable them to support mothers to successfully establish and maintain breastfeeding.
	2.	Understand the importance of human milk and breastfeeding to the health and wellbeing outcomes of mothers, babies and the wider family.
Theme 2: Support infant feeding	3.	Have an understanding of infant feeding culture within the UK and the various influences and constraints which impact on women's infant feeding decisions.
	4.	Be able to apply their knowledge and understanding of the physiology of lactation to support women to get breastfeeding off to a good start.
	5.	Be able to apply their knowledge of physiology and the principle of reciprocity to support mothers to keep their babies close and respond to their cues for feeding, love and comfort.
	6.	Have the knowledge and skills to support mothers and babies to maximise breastmilk and breastfeeding, to continue to breastfeed for as long as they wish and to introduce solid foods at an appropriate time.
	7.	Be able to support parents who formula feed to do so responsively and as safely as possible.
	8.	Understand the importance of the WHO International Code of Marketing of Breastmilk Substitutes and subsequent WHA resolutions (the Code) and how it impacts on practice.
Theme 3: Support close and loving relationships	9.	Develop an understanding of the importance of secure mother-infant attachment and the impact this has on their health and emotional wellbeing.
	10.	Be able to apply their knowledge of attachment theory to promote and encourage close and loving relationships between babies, their mothers and families, irrespective of their feeding method.
Theme 4: Managing the challenges	11.	Be able to apply their knowledge of the physiology of lactation and infant feeding to support effective management of challenges which may arise at any time during breastfeeding.
	12.	Have an understanding of the special circumstances which can affect lactation and breastfeeding (e.g. when mother and baby are separated, including preterm and sick infants) and be able to support mothers to overcome the challenges.
	13.	Draw on their knowledge and understanding of the wider social, cultural and political influences which undermine breastfeeding, to promote, support and protect breastfeeding within their sphere of practice.
Theme 5: Promote positive communication	14.	Have an understanding of the principles of effective communication and current thinking around public health promotion strategies and approaches.

(Continued)

Table 1.4 (Continued)

Theme	Learning outcomes	
	15.	Be able to apply their knowledge of effective communication to initiate sensitive, compassionate, mother-centred conversations with pregnant women and new mothers.
	16.	Have the knowledge and skills to access the evidence-based information that underpins infant feeding practice and know how to keep up-to-date (e.g. e-alerts, research summaries).

Source: www.unicef.org.uk/babyfriendly

In addition to developing effective communication styles and supporting parents to develop close and loving relationships, the education standards still include fundamental and basic knowledge about the normal anatomy of the breast, the physiology of lactation and the practical skills of breastfeeding, incorporating research-based evidence and consideration of the psycho-social factors that influence successful breastfeeding.

In a single-site case study in one of the first BFI-accredited pre-registration midwifery programmes in the UK, Pollard (2010) stated that student midwives reported feeling theoretically prepared for practice-based placements for their level of education and graduates of the programme also reported feeling confident at the point of registration to support and advise breastfeeding mothers. She also found that the accreditation process promoted a consistent approach to teaching and learning strategies, as well as content, within the curriculum. Furthermore, students believed it enhanced their employability prospects.

Global and national strategies

The WHO Code

The WHO (1981) developed the *International Code of Marketing of Breast-milk Substitutes*, known as the 'Code', to protect and promote breastfeeding and ensure the proper use of breastmilk substitutes. It is a World Health Assembly (WHA) resolution aimed at tackling a global health problem. Some of the requirements are:

- All formula milk labels should state the benefits of breastfeeding and the risks of formula feeding.
- There should be no promotion of breastmilk substitutes (this includes follow-on formulas and any solid foods or drinks sold for infants younger than the age of six months).
- No free samples of breastmilk substitutes are to be given to pregnant women.
- No free samples or subsidised substitutes are to be given to health workers or healthcare facilities.
- There should be no gifts for healthcare workers.
- Labels on products should not idealise formula feeding and should be written in an appropriate language.
- All information for healthcare workers should be factual and scientific.

It has been suggested that the Code removes choice from mothers, but instead the Code aims to improve choice by ensuring that advertising provides factual information for mothers on which to base their choices rather than biased information to sell a product. Although formula milk companies state on their products that breast milk is best, they do not provide information on the dangers of not breastfeeding. They also use persuasive language to suggest that formula milk is as 'good' as breastmilk when this is not possible.

The aim of adhering to the Code is to provide mothers with evidence-based information so they can make an informed choice about infant feeding and to protect against misleading marketing. Marketing activities of artificial milk companies and hospital practices have been identified as major reasons for the decline in breastfeeding. It is important that healthcare professionals do not accept gifts or samples from formula milk companies (which often include pens, diary covers, calendars and obstetric calculators), as these products are part of the marketing strategy, and accepting them suggests that healthcare professionals are endorsing the product.

However, if a mother chooses to formula feed her infant, all healthcare professionals should be equipped with up-to-date, factual and scientific information about the artificial milks available. Material available in healthcare journals is often intended for marketing purposes and therefore does not give all the facts. Healthcare workers must be objective when supporting mothers with formula feeding, should ensure information provided is evidence-based and should not promote one brand over another (NMC, 2015).

The Code was not fully adopted by the UK in law; instead, the government passed the *1995 Infant Formula and Follow-on Formula Regulations*. In 2007, the UK Minister for Public Health established a review of the *Infant Formula and Follow-on Formula Regulations* to reduce the confusion for parents between infant formula during the first months of life and follow-on formula for infants aged six months and older. They made the following recommendations:

- Manufacturers should make changes to advertising to make it clear that follow-on formula is intended for infants older than six months by clearly representing the age of the infants in the adverts.
- Any problems encountered with the enforcement of the regulations should be addressed accordingly.

In 2020 regulations governing the composition and marketing of infant milks changed and manufacturers of infant formula, follow-on formula and infant milks marketed as foods for special medical purposes must comply. To date the UK only includes some of the Code and does not cover inappropriate marketing of foods for use before age six months even though the introduction of solid food is recommended from six months of age (DHSC, 2022). There continues to be no regulations for the composition, marketing and or labelling of milks marketed for children older than 12 months of age ('growing up' or 'toddler' milks). Further detail can be accessed at www.bflg-uk.org.

Despite this, many healthcare settings that work to promote, protect and support breastfeeding and reduce inappropriate breastmilk substitute marketing have adopted the Code as part of their professional standards. Other professional and lay organisations have done the same, for example:

- UNICEF UK Baby Friendly Initiative.
- Baby Milk Action (BMA).
- International Baby Food Action Network (IBFAN).
- *Breastfeeding Manifesto* (BFM).
- Baby Feeding Law Group (BFLG, n.d.).

In February 2023 *The Lancet* launched a series on breastfeeding focusing on the power, reach and influence of commercial milk formula marketing practices. The three articles (Baker *et al.*, 2023; Pérez-Escamilla *et al.*, 2023; Rollins *et al.*, 2023) explore how normal infant feeding behaviours are framed as a reason to introduce formula milk by formula milk companies playing on mothers', families' and professionals' concerns (such as insufficient breastmilk, crying, fussiness and poor sleep) and confidence, undermining breastfeeding. The authors demonstrate a lack of evidence and unsubstantiated claims by manufacturers on the benefits of formula milk as well as the impact of the promotion of progression formula milk or products targeted at small babies that builds brand loyalty but negatively impacts on lifelong health and development and undermines the International Code of Breastmilk Substitutes. Instead of using the term 'breastmilk substitute', the authors use the term 'commercial milk formula' to clarify formula milk is artificial and a processed product to avoid the misconception that there is equivalence. They describe the increase in sales of formula milk across the world and the influence of marketing strategies on family health, policy and how it has changed the infant feeding 'ecosystem'. The authors identify breastfeeding success as a collective responsibility, not just the responsibility of the mother, and is dependent on multifaceted policy and society response. They call for governments to take action to address the imbalance in power between commercial interests and the needs and health of mothers and infants. A video of the launch of *The Lancet* series can be found on the WHO's website (www.who.int).

The Innocenti Declaration

The *Innocenti Declaration on the Protection, Promotion and Support of Breastfeeding* (WHO, 1990) was developed by WHO and UNICEF policy makers in 1990 and adopted in the UK and many other countries. It acknowledged the importance of exclusive breastfeeding for the first six months of life and its continuance thereafter alongside the introduction of solid foods. At the time it was apparent that there needed to be a change in some countries away from a bottle-feeding culture to a breastfeeding culture, which could only be achieved by removing obstacles to breastfeeding within healthcare systems, the workplace and society in general and, in doing so, increasing women's confidence in their ability to breastfeed. The declaration made the following recommendations:

- Women should be adequately nourished.
- Women should have access to family planning services to increase birth intervals and improve their health.
- All governments should develop a national breastfeeding policy and set appropriate targets that can be monitored.
- Breastfeeding policies should be integrated into other health and development policies.
- All governments should train healthcare staff to be able to implement the policies.
- National breastfeeding advisers should be appointed.
- Healthcare facilities should adhere to the WHO/UNICEF *Ten Steps to Successful Breastfeeding*.
- All governments should take cognisance of the *International Code of Marketing of Breast-milk Substitutes* and the WHA resolutions.
- All governments should enact legislation to protect breastfeeding mothers.

Activity

It is interesting to see how far the UK has come since the *Innocenti Declaration* in 1990. Identify some of the more recent and relevant policy documents that have recognised the need to promote breastfeeding to reduce health inequalities in your country of practice.

The UNICEF UK BFI (2016a) put out a call for action for the UK and devolved governments in UK to implement four key actions:

1 Develop a National Infant Feeding Board in each of the four nations to develop a National Infant Feeding Strategy and implementation plan.
2 Include actions to promote, protect and support breastfeeding in all policy areas where breastfeeding has an impact.
3 Implement evidence-based initiatives that support breastfeeding including UNICEF UK BFI across all maternity, health visiting, neonatal and children's centre services.
4 Protect the public from harmful commercial interests by adopting the Code.

The following year The Global Breastfeeding Collective (2017), a WHO and UNICEF initiative, identified seven policy action priorities with an indicator and target to be achieved by 2030 at national and global levels:

1 Funding: Increase investment in programmes that promote, protect and support breastfeeding.
2 Fully implement the Code with legislation and effective enforcement.
3 Maternity protection in the workplace: Provide paid maternity leave and workplace policies.
4 Implement the Ten Steps to Successful Breastfeeding in maternity facilities.
5 Improve access to skilled breastfeeding counselling in healthcare facilities.
6 Develop community support programmes.
7 Use monitoring systems to track progress on policies, programmes and funding.

Activity

Locate your local breastfeeding strategy and critically evaluate it to see if it reflects the 2017 UNICEF UK BFI standards.

- Have local breastfeeding targets been set?
- How are breastfeeding rates monitored?

Breastfeeding in public

Women have consistently reported negative attitudes and sometimes abuse directed at them when breastfeeding in public, and on occasion they have been removed from public areas or transport. In 2005, The Breastfeeding (Scotland) Act was passed, which made it an offence to prevent a person feeding milk by bottle or breast to an infant in a public place where the infant is legally entitled to be. Milk referred to breast, formula or cow's milk. Anyone who deliberately prevents a child being breast or bottle fed is guilty of an offence that could result in a fine. It was also intended that the Act would encourage, support and promote breastfeeding in Scotland by addressing negative attitudes.

Following this, in April 2009, the UK government presented an Equality Bill proposing that it was unlawful to prevent a woman from breastfeeding her baby in public. It was referred to as 'maternity' discrimination, which caused some confusion initially as this may only relate to six months before or after the birth and would therefore possibly not legally protect mothers breastfeeding for six months and beyond. It was amended to clarify that it meant mothers breastfeeding at any time (*The Equality Act*, 2010).

Despite legislation, the *Scottish Maternal and Infant Nutrition Survey* (SG, 2017) found 3 per cent of respondents reported being asked not to breastfeed or stop breastfeeding in a variety places, including NHS facilities.

Concluding comments

It is clear from the evidence that breastfeeding is essential in reducing health inequalities in mothers and infants in the UK. Despite this, mothers continue to face barriers that either discourage them from commencing breastfeeding or lead to early cessation of breastfeeding. Healthcare professionals need to be aware of the challenges mothers face in society and be equipped with the knowledge and skills to support them to overcome these barriers and confidently provide consistent information to manage these challenges as they arise. There is a wealth of information available to both mothers and healthcare professionals today, particularly online, and access is now available to most people. Developing knowledge and skills to support breastfeeding mothers is discussed further in Chapter 12.

Practice questions

1 In your area of practice, how and when do you inform mothers about the benefits of breastfeeding and the dangers of not breastfeeding?
2 Are there services targeted at the socio-economic characteristics of mothers in your area of practice? How do women find out about available services?
3 Go back and read the Ten Steps in Table 1.2 and the BFI Standards in Table 1.3. Are these standards implemented in your area of practice? If not, why not?
4 In relation to marketing of formula milk, does your area of practice comply with the WHO Code? How do you find out about new information on formula milk, and how do you share it with mothers?
5 Has your university integrated the UNICEF UK BFI university learning outcomes (see Table 1.3) into pre-registration programmes?
6 If yes, what difference do you think this has made to your practice?
7 If no, what advantages do you think accreditation would bring to the programmes and to practice?

Resources

- Baby Feeding Law Group (BFLG, n.d.)
  www.bflg-uk.org/

- Baby Milk Action (BMA)
  www.babymilkaction.org/

- Healthy Start
  www.healthystart.nhs.uk/

- UNICEF UK Baby Friendly Initiative
  www.unicef.org.uk/babyfriendly/

2   Building relationships

- Learning outcomes
- Brain development and importance of love and nurture
- Responsive care
- Responsive feeding
- Concluding comments
- Reflective questions
- Resources

There has been an increase in neuroscience research on the long-term impact of parental relationships on brain development in unborn infants and during the early years. This chapter will enable readers to develop an understanding of secure mother–infant attachment and the impact this has on their health and emotional well-being. Although attachments will form with other caregivers (e.g. the father), the focus of this chapter is on attachment theory to promote and encourage close and loving relationships between mother and infant.

Learning outcomes

By the end of this chapter, you will be able to:

- discuss the importance of love and nurture in brain development;
- support mothers to build confidence in their ability to feed and care for their infants; and
- provide advice for mothers to bottle-feed responsively.

Mapping to UNICEF UK BFI Education learning outcomes (2019a)
  By the end of the programme, students will:

Theme		Learning outcomes
Theme 2: Support infant feeding	5.	Be able to apply their knowledge of physiology and the principle of reciprocity to support mothers to keep their babies close and respond to their cues for feeding, love and comfort.

DOI: 10.4324/9781003282341-2

Theme		Learning outcomes
	7.	Be able to support parents who formula feed to do so responsively and as safely as possible.
Theme 3: Support close and loving relationships	9.	Develop an understanding of the importance of secure mother-infant attachment and the impact this has on their health and emotional wellbeing.
	10.	Be able to apply their knowledge of attachment theory to promote and encourage close and loving relationships between babies, their mothers and families, irrespective of their feeding method.

Brain development and the importance of love and nurture

The mother–infant relationship begins in pregnancy, so it is important that healthcare professionals encourage and support women to maximise opportunities to connect with their baby. This can be achieved by discussing the development stages of the fetus, including brain development and ability to hear and sense moods. Stress in pregnancy and the effect on fetal development should also be discussed, as well as ways to minimise it. Cortisol is produced in response to stress and prolonged exposure to high levels of cortisol may have a negative effect on growth and brain development of the fetus (Graignic-Philippe *et al.*, 2014; Fitzgerald *et al.*, 2020). Healthcare professionals should advise mothers on strategies that will increase oxytocin levels to counteract the effect of cortisol.

UNICEF UK BFI facilitate a course and have a number of resources for healthcare professionals to support close and loving relationships between parents and babies (www.unicef.org.uk/babyfriendly). In the guide for parents 'Building a Happy Baby', UNICEF UK BFI (2021) recommends the following ways a mother, partner and siblings can make a connection with the baby and also create a positive environment for brain development:

- During pregnancy, talking, reading, stroking and playing music.
- Skin-to skin contact after birth.
- Keeping the baby close and cuddle skin to skin in early days.
- Responding to the baby's cues for food and comfort.
- Looking face to face, talking and listening to the baby.

Brain development begins in pregnancy and continues at a rapid rate in the first two years until adolescence and beyond. By the age of six years, the brain has developed to 90 per cent of adult capacity (Stiles and Jernigan, 2010). Information is processed by the formation of networks of neurons which communicate with each other using electrical and chemical signals and form the basis of learning and memory. Messages are passed between neurons at connections called synapses. At birth there are billions of neurons that immediately start to make connections or synapses between the neurons as a result of interaction. The more they are triggered by social interaction, in particular with the parents, the more they develop.

The growth of the brain is expeditious; it weighs approximately 400 grams at birth and by one year of age approximately 1000 grams due to the density of neural

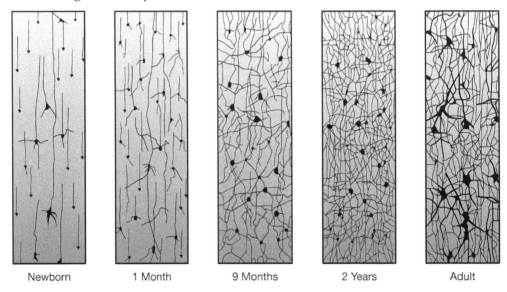

Figure 2.1 Infant brain development (synapse density over time)

Source: Adapted from Corel, JL. The postnatal development of the human cerebral cortex. Cambridge, MA: Harvard University Press; 1975.

connections (Figure 2.1). Synapses are formed at a faster rate during the first three years than any other time in life, and by age three years, it has reached 80 per cent of its adult volume (see Table 2.1). Brain development is a delicate interplay of genetic and environmental factors. In early development genes impact on the structure and organisation of neurons but the fine-tuning of development and stimulation of neural development is reliant on experiences and environment. For example, language development – the more the infant is spoken to the greater the stimulation and activation of the synapses between neurons. Repeated use increases the strength of the synapse, which in turn strengthens cognitive ability. If they are not activated regularly, they will be weak or lost. Infants have an under-developed neocortex (responsible for rational thought and creative thinking), so their behaviour is controlled by the limbic system (which controls basic emotion, fear and pleasure) via the autonomic nervous system, hormonal system and muscular (somatic) system. This means they cannot rationalise their feelings of fear or distress and need their parents to be caring and provide comfort to enable them to cope with emotions. If parents do not provide this comfort and help infants to learn to manage these feelings in early childhood, the infant will remain in a state of hyper-arousal, resulting in prolonged high levels of cortisol. Evidence suggests this could have long-term impact on memory and reduced cognition, attention deficit and behavioural problems (Letourneau *et al.*, 2011). Parents can comfort their babies and reduce cortisol levels by keeping the bay close, cuddling and comforting them when they cry and not leaving them alone, using skin-to-skin contact and talking to and touching the baby.

If an infant has been exposed to prolonged stress and high cortisol levels in pregnancy, prolonged and frequent skin-to-skin contact will help to calm both mother and

Table 2.1 Early brain development

Trimester 1	The neural tube forms and continues to change, eventually becoming the brain and spinal cord. The first neurons and synapses begin to develop and allow the fetus to move and provide the brain with sensory input to promote development.
Trimester 2	The cerebral cortex increases in thickness, complexity and synapse formation. Myelination of some neurons begins, which allows faster processing of information.
Trimester 3	Reflexes such as fetal breathing and responses to external stimuli become more regular (following the development of the cerebral cortex), as well as early learning.
Year 1	Newborns can recognise human faces, can discriminate between happy and sad expressions and can recognise their mothers' voices. The cerebellum triples in size, associated to the rapid development of motor skills. Visual areas of the cortex grow. There is growth in the hippocampus, the limbic structure related to recognition memory. Language circuits in the frontal and temporal lobes become consolidated in the first year (dependent on exposure to speech).
Year 2	There are major changes in language areas, including increases in synapses and connections, resulting in an increase in vocabulary. There is a major increase in the rate of myelination to improve speed and ability to perform complex tasks. Higher-order cognitive abilities like self-awareness develop; infants are now more aware of their own emotions and intentions.
Year 3	The synaptic density in the prefrontal cortex reaches its peak. Cognitive abilities are improved and consolidated. Children have the ability to use past experiences to interpret present events and demonstrate an understanding of cause and effect.

Adapted from www.urbanchildinstitute.org (accessed October 2022)

infant and increase levels of oxytocin. High levels of oxytocin produced when mother and infant are in close contact affect receptor sites in the brain, encouraging right-brain (random, subjective, holistic and intuitive) dominance, which further enhances the relationship and attachment between mother and infant. Attachment experiences in the first two years are known to directly influence the development of the right brain. This includes traumatic experiences with a caregiver, which can have a negative impact on the child's sense of security, ability to cope with stress and sense of self (Schore, 2001).

The role of cortisol and oxytocin

Cortisol is produced by the adrenal gland, but release is controlled by the hypothalamus. Corticotropin-releasing hormone triggers cells in the anterior pituitary to secrete adrenocorticotropic hormone (ACTH), which is transported via the blood stream to the adrenal cortex and stimulates synthesis of cortisol. Whilst cortisol is required for lactation, high levels are associated with a delay in lactogenesis. There is also a suggestion that cortisol in breastmilk may reduce immunoglobulin-producing cells (Wambach and Riordan, 2016).

Cortisol levels of mother and infant are similar, and prolonged exposure to cortisol has been associated with reduced cognition and memory, attention problems and behavioural difficulties in children and postpartum depression in mothers (Letourneau *et al.*, 2011). In addition, infants born to mothers with high cortisol levels demonstrate more crying and negative facial expressions. In a study of 63 breastfeeding mothers, Handlin *et al.* (2009) found ACTH and cortisol levels fell significantly during breastfeeding. They demonstrated a significant negative relationship between oxytocin and ACTH levels and a significant positive relationship between ACTH and cortisol levels, concluding that breastfeeding and skin-to-skin contact are associated to reduced production of ACTH and reduced cortisol levels.

Oxytocin is often referred to as the 'love hormone'. It is known that a reduction in cortisol levels results in a sense of calmness, lower blood pressure, reduced anxiety and promotion of maternal behaviour (Moberg, 2003; Uvnäs-Moberg *et al.*, 2020). As discussed further in Chapter 3, oxytocin is essential for the 'let-down' reflex and milk ejection which is triggered by the mother's seeing, hearing, touching or smelling her infant, and with increasing age, it can be triggered by just thinking about the infant (Moberg, 2003).

Responsive care

The theory of attachment was developed by John Bowlby (1982) to describe the bond from a child towards their parent or primary caregiver to promote survival. Bowlby suggested that the infant's ability to cope with stress was directly related to maternal behaviour. Prior and Glaser (2006) describe four phases of the development of attachment:

- Phase 1: Birth to 8 weeks (initial pre-attachment)
  The infant uses behaviours such as smiling, crying and grasping to attract attention. The parents learn how to recognise the cues and the interaction forms the basis of attachment.
- Phase 2: 8 weeks to 6 months (attachment in the making)
  Infant distinguishes between adults and focuses on the parents.
- Phase 3: 6–36 months (clear-cut attachment)
  Infant demonstrates preference for primary caregiver and demonstrates anxiety and distress if separated.
- Phase 4: 36 months onwards (goal-corrected partnership)
  Infant becomes less distressed at separation from care givers and uses language to express their needs.

Consistent responsive care and interaction is essential to build a strong relationship that will enhance an infant's ongoing development. Infants quickly learn whether their parents will care for them and make them feel secure in their environment. In the past mothers were advised to leave a baby to cry and not to keep picking them up as they would become 'spoiled'. However, it is clear from the evidence that this has a detrimental effect on development as infants cannot manage the stress of separation. The resulting high level of cortisol is thought to result in a state of hyper-arousal and dissociation (or submission and resignation to the inevitable danger). Schore (2001) suggests if this state becomes chronic, it has a negative effect on the limbic structures, brain growth and development, along the lines of 'if you don't use it, you lose it'.

The RCM (2020) identify the key components of early parenting as the sharing and regulation of emotions and behaviour (attunement); parent and infant taking turn to initiate, sustain and stop interactions (reciprocity); parent's mirroring emotion so the infant knows the parent understands (marked mirroring); helping the infant to manage emotion by communicating empathy using touch or speech (containment) and parent's ability to learn to understand the infant's feelings and individual traits (reflective function) (Figure 2.2).

There are a number of factors that can have a negative impact on building close and loving relationships such as domestic abuse, substance misuse and mental health problems. NICE (2018a) developed the public health guideline '*Social and emotional wellbeing: Early years. Recommendation 3 antenatal and postnatal home visiting for vulnerable children and their families*' aimed at midwives, health visitors and early years services.

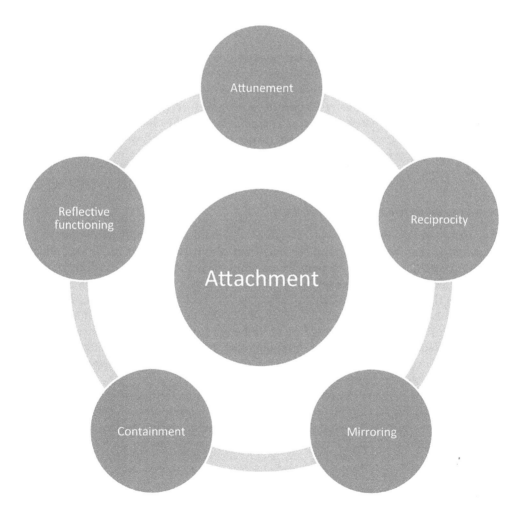

Figure 2.2 Components of a positive relationship

Source: RCM (2020), Key aspects of early parenting.

They recommend a series of intensive home visits for parents, who need additional support, to ensure healthy development of the infant. The goal of the visits should be in relation to:

- maternal sensitivity to her infant's needs;
- the mother–infant relationship;
- home learning – speech, language and communication skills;
- parenting skills and practice; and
- development of father–infant relationship.

Some of the interventions they recommend include baby massage and video interaction guidance. The National Institute for Health and Clinical Excellence (NICE) also emphasise the importance of partnership working with other early years practitioners to promote coordinated support.

Responsive feeding

Infant feeding is a learning process for both the parents and the infant and can be a daunting experience, whether breastfeeding or bottle feeding. Many parents have had no previous experience and feel anxious about the responsibility. Habron *et al.* (2013, pp. 141–149) describe responsive feeding as 'a reciprocal relationship between an infant or child and his or her caregiver that is characterised by the child communicating feelings of hunger and satiety through verbal or nonverbal cues, followed by an immediate response from the caregiver'. Responsive breastfeeding is discussed further in Chapters 3, 4 and 5.

Supporting mothers to bottle feed responsively

For a variety of reasons discussed throughout this book, some mothers choose to bottle feed rather than breastfeed, and these mothers also need support to build confidence and maximise the benefits of responsive care and feeding discussed. Responsive care is thought to prevent raised cortisol levels (Letourneau *et al.*, 2011). Continuity in who bottle feeds the infant, particularly in early days, is crucial to build a close, loving and reciprocal relationship. Family and friends often offer to bottle feed the infant to give the mother a rest; however, it would be more helpful to support the mother with more practical help such as housework or shopping to let the mother spend time with her baby to learn feeding cues and recognise behaviour traits so she can respond appropriately and enable the baby to feel secure.

Whilst there is limited evidence about responsive formula feeding, it is possible to overfeed a formula fed infant. Current evidence suggests that nonresponsive feeding is associated with child obesity, but Hurley *et al.* (2011) suggest more research is needed, particularly in high-income countries. UNICEF UK BFI recommend that parents are advised to

- respond to cues that their baby is hungry;
- invite the baby to draw on the teat rather than pushing in to the mouth;
- pace the feed so the baby isn't encouraged to take more than is required; and
- recognise when the baby has had enough.

Formula feeding is considered in further detail in Chapter 9.

Concluding comments

Healthcare professionals must understand early brain development and the impact of a close and loving relationship on the future behaviour, success and resilience of a child. There is a delicate interplay between genetic and environmental factors and children are vulnerable to negative influences, particularly in the prenatal and early years. To ensure this time of opportunity is embraced, parents must be supported to maximise developmental opportunities that cannot be re-claimed – 'if you don't use it, you lose it'.

Reflective questions

1 How do you support parents to start building a relationship with their baby during pregnancy?
2 Do you discuss the importance of avoiding stress in pregnancy?
3 How do you support mothers to bottle feed responsively?

Resources

- NHS Pregnancy Week-by-Week
  www.nhs.uk/pregnancy/week-by-week

- The Basics of Brain Development by J. Stiles and T. Jernigan:
  www.ncbi.nlm.nih.gov/pmc/articles/PMC2989000

- UNICEF BFI (201b) Responsive Feeding: Supporting Close and Loving Relationships
  www.unicef.org.uk/babyfriendly

3 Anatomy and physiology of lactation

- Learning outcomes
- Relevant anatomy and physiology
- The physiology of lactation
- Properties of breastmilk
- Neonatal adaptation to life
- Concluding comments
- True or false quiz
- Further reading

It is essential for healthcare professionals to have a sound knowledge of the external and internal anatomy of the breast, as well as the physiology of lactation, to support mothers effectively to feel confident about positioning and attachment, hand expression and the management of common problems. This chapter begins with an introduction to breast development in puberty, pregnancy and lactation and goes on to discuss the anatomy of the breast and the physiology of lactation. The first chapter identified the benefits of breastmilk in promoting good health and reducing health inequalities, whilst Chapter 2 discussed the importance of building a mother's self-confidence in her ability to feed and care for her baby. This chapter moves on to discuss the properties of breastmilk that make it the ideal form of nutrition for human infants. Finally, production of breastmilk will not be continued without effective removal of breastmilk from the breast; therefore, it is crucial that healthcare professionals have a clear understanding of the mechanism of suckling and adaptation to life to teach mothers to recognise appropriate feeding behaviour.

Learning outcomes

By the end of this chapter, you will be able to:

- understand breast development in pregnancy and lactation;
- describe the anatomy of the breast;
- understand the physiology of lactation;
- describe the constituents and value of colostrum and breastmilk; and
- demonstrate an understanding of the mechanism of infant suckling.

DOI: 10.4324/9781003282341-3

Mapping to UNICEF Baby Friendly Initiative (BFI) Education learning outcomes (2019a)

By the end of the programme, students will:

Theme		Learning outcomes
Theme 1: Understand breastfeeding	1.	Have sufficient knowledge of anatomy of the breast and physiology of lactation to enable them to support mothers to successfully establish and maintain breastfeeding.
	2.	Understand the importance of human milk and breastfeeding to the health and wellbeing outcomes of mothers, babies and the wider family.
Theme 2: Support infant feeding	4.	Be able to apply their knowledge and understanding of the physiology of lactation to support women to get breastfeeding off to a good start.
	5.	Be able to apply their knowledge of physiology and the principle of reciprocity to support mothers to keep their babies close and respond to their cues for feeding, love and comfort.
	6.	Have the knowledge and skills to support mothers and babies to maximise breastmilk and breastfeeding, to continue to breastfeed for as long as they wish and to introduce solid foods at an appropriate time.

Relevant anatomy and physiology

Mammogenesis

'Mammogenesis' is the term used for the development of the mammary glands or breasts, which occurs in five stages:

- embryogenesis;
- puberty;
- pregnancy;
- lactation; and
- involution

Embryogenesis

Mammogenesis or breast development begins at about the fourth week of gestation in both male and female fetuses. By 12 to 16 weeks, the development of the nipple and areola is evident. The lactiferous ducts open into the mammary pit, which elevates to become the nipple and areola. After birth some neonates born at term secrete a fluid referred to as 'witch's milk' (not known in premature infants) due to the influence of the maternal hormones associated with milk production. This should not be expressed as it can be painful and lead to infection (Dayal *et al.*, 2016).

Interesting fact

Witch's milk is present in both sexes and can continue up to two months of age. The name 'witch's milk' is derived from folklore, in which it was thought to be a source of nourishment for witches' familiars and was taken from sleeping babies.

Puberty

There is no further breast development until puberty, when increasing levels of oestrogen and progesterone lead to growth of lactiferous ducts, alveoli, the nipples and the areolas. The increase in breast size is due to the deposition of adipose tissue (Geddes, 2007a; Geddes *et al.*, 2021).

Pregnancy and lactogenesis

For many women breast changes can be one of the first signs of pregnancy. At about the sixth week of pregnancy, oestrogen promotes the growth of the lactiferous ducts, while progesterone, prolactin and human placental lactogen (HPL) lead to proliferation and enlargement of the alveoli; women describe a 'tingling' sensation, sensitivity and heaviness of their breasts (Pollard, 2023). With the increasing blood supply, veins become visible on the surface of the breasts. At 12 weeks, there is greater pigmentation to the areola and nipples due to increased melanocytes, and they become red/brown in colour. The *Montgomery's tubercles* also become more prominent and begin to excrete a serous lubricant to protect the nipple and areola. At approximately 16 weeks, colostrum is produced (lactogenesis I) under the influence of prolactin and HPL, but complete milk production is suppressed by the increased levels of oestrogen and progesterone. However, some women may find they secrete a clear fluid prior to this. At approximately 24 weeks, the secondary areola is formed around the areola.

Involution

Involution occurs when weaning takes place and milk is no longer removed from the breast. Prolactin production is no longer stimulated and there is milk stasis and subsequent build-up of feedback inhibitor of lactation (FIL), which inhibits further milk synthesis. The secretory epithelial cells die (apoptosis), are reabsorbed and the breasts return to the pre-pregnant size by approximately 15 months (Kent, 2007).

As the infant is introduced to solid food, the composition and volume of breastmilk changes from an average of 759 ml per day to 95–315 ml per day at 15 months of age. There is also a decrease in glucose and minerals and an increase in fat, lactose, protein and sodium (Kent, 2007), giving the milk a more salty taste.

External structure of the breast

The breasts, or mammary glands, are hemispherical in shape and normally depicted with an axillary tail and are situated on each side of the anterior chest wall (Figure 3.1).

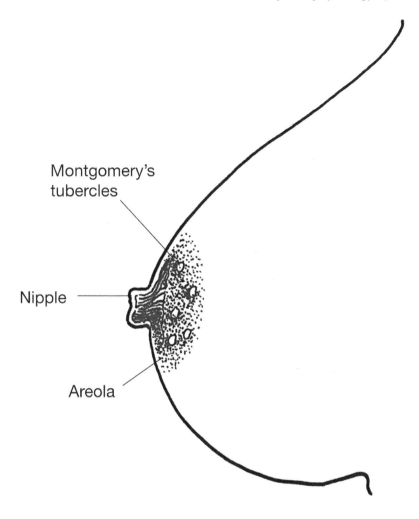

Figure 3.1 The external structure of the breast

They extend from the second to the sixth rib, from the sternum to the axilla (the *tail of Spence*), over the pectoralis muscles. However, more recently Teplica *et al.* (2022) have argued against the existence of the tail of Spence. They conducted pinch testing and topographic mapping of 316 people in preparation for breast and gynecomastia surgery. Instead, they suggest, the outer half of the chest is defined by three adipose structures – an axillary mound, the primary breast mound and a previously unnamed lateral chest wall tail with no anatomic evidence of an 'axillary tail' of fat extending from the breast to axilla.

The breasts are supported by fibrous connective tissue called Cooper's ligaments. Each mother's breasts vary in size; this is determined by the amount of fatty tissue, not glandular tissue. Size is not an indicator of milk storage capacity. Each mother's storage capacity is variable but, despite this, over a 24-hour period, all lactating mothers produce a similar amount of breastmilk (average 750–800 ml/24 hours) (Kent *et al.*, 2006; Geddes *et al.*, 2021). The main difference is noted in feeding patterns, and mothers with lower storage capacity breastfeed more frequently than those with higher storage capacity, thus supporting the argument for responsive feeding. Geddes *et al.* (2021) suggested milk production for mothers of male infants is greater as they consume on average 80–100 ml more breastmilk per day.

At the midpoint on the exterior surface lies the *areola*, a pigmented area. On average the areola measures 15 mm in diameter; however, every woman's areola differs in size and colour. The Montgomery's tubercles open into the areola and secrete a protective oily secretion to lubricate the nipple during breastfeeding. The dark area of the areola is thought to assist the baby to find the nipple at birth, and the scent is also thought to help attract the infant to suckle at the breast (Schaal *et al.*, 2005; Geddes, 2007a; Geddes *et al.*, 2021). The *nipple* is a sensitive erectile structure that contains smooth muscle, collagen and elastic connective tissue found in both circular and radial formations. During pregnancy it increases in size and length. Erection of the nipple is stimulated by tactile and autonomic sympathetic responses. It lies at the centre of the areola, from where breastmilk is ejected on demand. Stimulation of the nipple causes milk ejection via the hypothalamus, which stimulates oxytocin release from the posterior pituitary gland (Uvnäs-Moberg *et al.*, 2020).

Internal structure of the lactating breast

Until recently, the internal anatomy of the breast was based on wax casts from dissections of cadavers by Sir Astley Cooper in 1840. In 2005, Ramsay *et al.* conducted research using ultrasound imaging and described a number of differences in the structure of the breast.

The *lactiferous ducts* were previously thought to lead to the lactiferous sinus; however, Ramsay *et al.* (2005) found that the ducts branched off within the *areola* approximately 5–8 mm from the nipple, closer to the nipple than previously thought, and did not demonstrate evidence of sinuses. The *lactiferous ducts* are small (mean diameter, 2 mm), superficial and easy to compress (Figure 3.2). The authors of this study suggest that the ducts are responsible for transportation of the milk rather than storage. They also found that the network of milk ducts is not homogeneous as previously suggested. Ramsay *et al.* (2005) found that there were 4–18 (average, 9) main milk ducts.

The breast is shaped by the fat and glandular tissue, which is inseparable except subcutaneously where there is only fat (Nickell and Skelton, 2005). The ratio of glandular to fat tissue increases to a ratio of 2:1 in the lactating breast compared with 1:1 in non-lactating women, and 65 per cent of the glandular tissue is located within 30 mm from the base of the nipple (Hilton, 2008).

Numerous *alveoli* (10–100) (Figure 3.3) cluster to form lobules, which are grouped into lobes. They are often described as being like a bunch of grapes. The alveoli consist of a single layer of the milk-producing *lactocytes* (*secretory epithelium*), which are surrounded by a network of capillaries. Lactocytes line the lumen of the alveoli and are cuboidal in shape if full and columnar if empty. They are connected to each other and regulate the composition of breastmilk for collection in the lumen of the

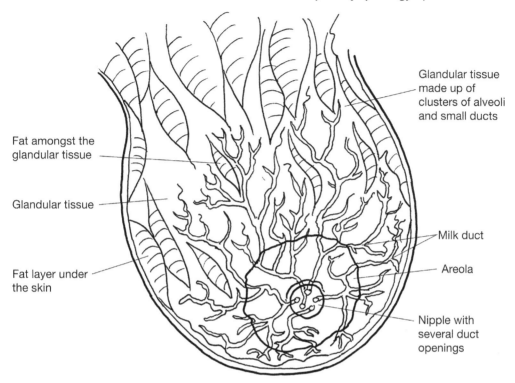

Glandular tissue made up of clusters of alveoli and small ducts

Fat amongst the glandular tissue

Glandular tissue

Fat layer under the skin

Milk duct

Areola

Nipple with several duct openings

Figure 3.2 The internal anatomy of the lactating breast
Source: Adapted from © UNICEF UK BFI.

alveoli. It is this shape or fullness of the lactocyte that controls synthesis of breast-milk. If the lactocyte becomes too full and the shape distorts, the prolactin receptor sites do not function, leading to decreased milk synthesis (van Veldhuizen-Staas, 2007). Once emptied, the lactocytes resume the normal columnar shape and milk synthesis can recommence. Tight junctions connect these cells and are closed in the first few days of lactation, preventing the passage of molecules through the space. The portion of the lactocytes facing the lumen is called the *apical surface*; the outer aspect is *basal*. Milk secretion occurs at the apical surface, whereas the basal aspect of the cell is responsible for the selection and synthesis of substrates from the blood (Geddes, 2007a).

Key fact

Breasts should be effectively emptied on a regular basis, either by suckling or expression, otherwise the shape of the lactocytes distorts, and milk production ceases.

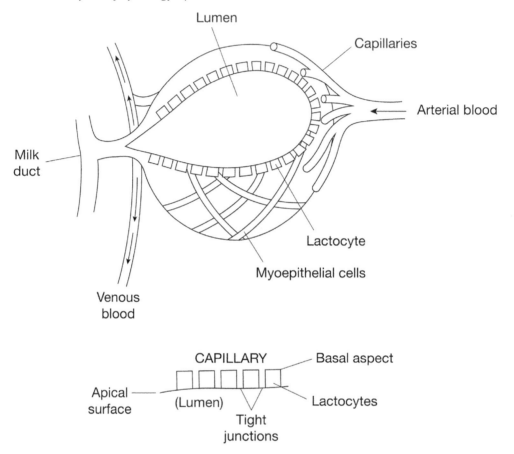

Figure 3.3 An alveolus
Source: Adapted from Berry *et al.* (2007).

The alveoli are surrounded by myoepithelial cells, which, under the influence of oxytocin, contract to expel the breastmilk from the lumen of the alveolus along the lactiferous ducts to the awaiting infant (Figure 3.4). Multiple milk ejections occur during a breastfeed or expression of milk, with a range of 0–9 ejections (Geddes, 2007a).

Blood, nerves and lymphatic system

The breasts are highly vascular; 60 per cent of the blood supply is via the internal mammary artery and 30 per cent via the lateral thoracic artery. Venous drainage is via the mammary and axillary veins. The lymphatic system drains excess fluid from the tissue spaces into the axillary nodes and mammary nodes (Geddes, 2007a).

The skin is supplied by branches of the thoracic nerves and the nipple and areola by the autonomic nervous system. The nerve supply is mainly from branches of the fourth, fifth and sixth intercostal nerves. The fourth intercostal nerve becomes superficial at the areola, where it divides into five branches. Trauma, such as breast surgery, to this nerve may lead to loss of sensation (Geddes, 2007b).

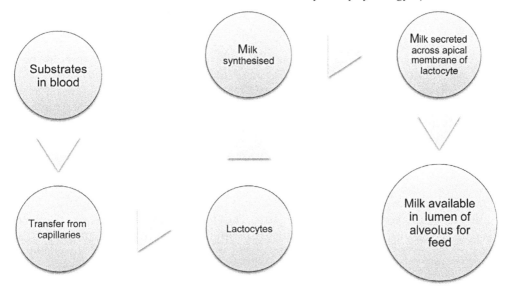

Figure 3.4 Pathway for the synthesis of breastmilk

The physiology of lactation

Lactogenesis is the initiation of milk production. There are three phases of lactogenesis. The first two phases are hormonally driven or *neuroendocrine* responses (interaction between the nervous system and the endocrine system) and occur whether the mother intends to breastfeed or not; the third is *autocrine* (a cell secretes a hormone chemical that acts on itself) or by local control.

Neuroendocrine control

Lactogenesis I is thought to occur at around 16 weeks' gestation when colostrum is produced by lactocytes under neuroendocrine control. Prolactin, although present during pregnancy, is inhibited by the increased levels of progesterone and oestrogen as well as HPL and prolactin-inhibiting factor (PIF), and therefore milk production is suppressed. However, some mothers may leak colostrum or choose to express colostrum from 36 weeks (see Chapter 7, 'Diabetes').

Lactogenesis II is the onset of milk production. It occurs following expulsion of the placenta and membranes, which results in a sudden drop in progesterone, oestrogen, HPL and PIF (neuroendocrine control). Prolactin levels increase and bind with prolactin receptors in the walls of the lactocytes, which are no longer deactivated by HPL and PIF, and begin milk synthesis. Skin-to-skin contact at birth with the baby stimulates the production of prolactin and oxytocin. Early and regular breastfeeding inhibits the production of PIF and stimulates production of prolactin. Mothers should be encouraged to commence breastfeeding as soon as possible following birth to stimulate milk production and to provide infants with colostrum (Czank *et al.*, 2007a).

Key fact

Lactogenesis II may be delayed in mothers with type 1 diabetes, possibly due to the initial imbalance in insulin levels required for lactation, and those with retained placental products due to prolonged production of progesterone. Therefore, prolonged skin-to-skin contact from birth should be encouraged for uninterrupted access to the breast. If the infant does not suckle, regular hand expression will be required to stimulate milk production.

Lactogenesis II commences 30–40 hours after birth, but mothers do not feel the milk 'coming in' until about 2–3 days after birth. The increase in milk production is associated with the closure of the tight junctions between the lactocytes (Czank *et al.*, 2007a).

Prolactin

Prolactin is the hormone essential in the establishment and maintenance of breastmilk production and is highest following the delivery of the placenta and membranes (200 µg g/l) but gradually reduces by six months postpartum (80 µg g/l) (Cox *et al.*, 1996). It is released into the blood from the anterior pituitary gland in responses to suckling or nipple stimulation and primes and stimulates the prolactin receptor sites on the walls of the lactocytes to synthesise milk (Czank *et al.*, 2007a) (Figure 3.5). The prolactin receptor sites regulate the secretion of breastmilk. When the alveoli are full of milk, the walls expand and change shape, affecting the prolactin receptor sites; ultimately, prolactin is unable to enter the cells, and the milk production rate decreases. As the milk is emptied from the alveolus, its normal shape is returned, and prolactin binds to the receptor site, increasing milk production (van Veldhuizen-Staas, 2007). Prolactin is also secreted during breastfeeding and is at its highest rate 45 minutes after a feed. Prolactin levels peak at night (circadian rhythm); therefore, night feeds must be encouraged to promote milk production.

Key fact

The prolactin receptor theory suggests that frequent milk removal in the early days increases the number of prolactin receptor sites 'switched on', thus improving milk production.

Oxytocin

Oxytocin is released from the posterior pituitary gland and stimulates contraction of the *myoepithelial cells* surrounding the alveoli to eject milk through the lactiferous ducts (see Figure 3.5). This is commonly referred to as the let-down, oxytocin or ejection reflex. It causes shortening of the lactiferous ducts to increase the intraductal mammary pressure and thus to facilitate milk ejection. Some women feel a 'tingling' sensation in the breast

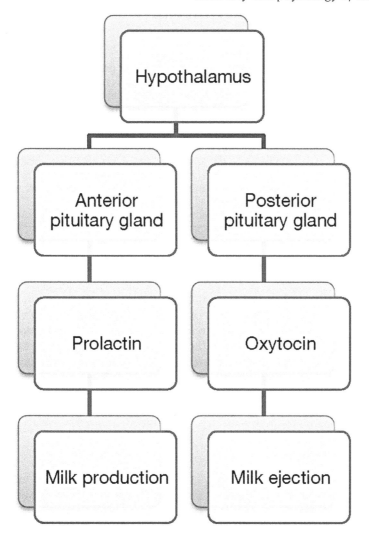

Figure 3.5 The neuroendocrine response

and uterine contractions with increased bleeding per vagina within the first few days after birth. Some also describe feeling thirsty, flushing and becoming sleepy. Oxytocin, often called the 'love hormone', reduces cortisol levels, resulting in a relaxing effect, reducing anxiety and blood pressure and promoting maternal behaviour (Moberg, 2003). The let-down reflex is controlled in the first few days following birth by the neonate suckling at the breast and by the mother seeing, touching, hearing and smelling her baby (Uvnäs-Moberg *et al.*, 2020). As the infant becomes older, the let-down reflex may be triggered by thinking about feeding the baby or hearing another baby cry. Ramsay *et al.* (2005) found that 75 per cent of breastfeeding mothers experience more than one let-down reflex per feed (average, 2.5) and that 33 per cent of infants end the feed after the first let-down reflex. The let-down reflex can, however, be inhibited by stress and anxiety.

Table 3.1 The influence of other hormones on lactation

Hormone	Function
Glucocorticoids	Essential for mammary development in pregnancy, onset of lactogenesis II and maintenance of lactogenesis (galactopoesis)
Growth hormone	Essential for the maintenance of lactation by regulating metabolism
Insulin	Ensures nutrients are readily available for milk synthesis
Placental lactogen	Produced by the placenta and stimulates mammary development and growth but is not involved in lactogenesis I or II
Progesterone	Inhibits lactogenesis II during pregnancy by suppressing the prolactin receptor sites in the lactocytes. Once lactation is established, progesterone has little effect on breastmilk supply and therefore the progesterone-only contraceptive pill may be used by breastfeeding mothers (Czank *et al.*, 2007a)
Thyroxin	Assists the breasts to be responsive to growth hormone and prolactin

It is thought that suckling in neonates is optimal at 45 minutes following birth and declines within two to three hours in line with the physiological reduction in neonatal adrenaline levels at birth. It is therefore important that mothers and infants are able to have skin-to-skin contact for a minimum of one hour following birth to encourage early feeding, which ensures that prolactin is released, leading to the commencement of lactogenesis II. Other factors thought to interfere with lactogenesis are retained placenta, Sheehan's syndrome or pituitary shock, breast surgery, type I diabetes, preterm delivery, obesity and stress. These issues are addressed in Chapters 7 and 8. Table 3.1 provides an overview of the influence of hormones on lactation.

Practice recommendations

- Encourage skin-to-skin contact for a minimum of one hour following birth.
- Encourage suckling at the breast as soon after birth as possible to stimulate production of prolactin.
- Encourage regular breastfeeding and promote night feeds when levels of prolactin are highest. If this is not possible, regular expression of breastmilk is required.
- Avoid separation of the mother and infant and promote 'rooming-in'.
- Create a relaxed environment for feeding or expressing because stress inhibits the release of oxytocin.

Autocrine control

Lactogenesis III indicates the autocrine regulation in which supply and demand regulate milk production. As well as the neuroendocrine response described earlier, milk supply is also controlled at the breast by milk removal through autocrine or local control. By studying milk production in goats, the Hannah Institute, Ayr, identified a whey protein called the Feedback Inhibitor of Lactation (FIL), secreted by the lactocytes, which regulates milk production at a local level (Wilde *et al.*, 1995; Knight *et al.*, 1998). As the alveoli distend, there is a build-up of FIL, and milk synthesis is inhibited (Figure 3.6). When the breastmilk

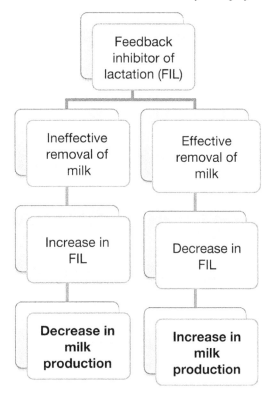

Figure 3.6 The autocrine or local response

is effectively removed and the concentrations of FIL reduce, milk synthesis resumes. This is a local mechanism and can occur in one or both breasts. It exerts a negative feedback response to inhibit milk production when there is ineffective removal of the breastmilk from the breast (Czank *et al.*, 2007a).

Key fact

If an infant is incorrectly attached to the breast or unable to remove the breastmilk from the breast, there will be a build-up of FIL, culminating in a reduced supply of breastmilk. This can be rectified by regular and effective emptying of the breast by correcting positioning and attachment or expressing breastmilk at regular intervals. See Chapter 4 for further information.

Practice recommendations

- Promote responsive feeding.
- Ensure correct positioning and attachment at the breast to facilitate effective removal of milk from the breast (see Chapter 4).

- Avoid supplementary feeds such as formula milk and water, as this will lead to irregular removal of milk and subsequent build-up of FIL and a decrease in milk supply.
- Increased stimulation of the breast through infant sucking or expression can lead to increased growth of secretory breast tissue and induce lactation in non-lactating women.

Properties of breastmilk

Colostrum

Colostrum is produced from approximately the 16th week of pregnancy (lactogenesis I) and is present and ready for birth. It develops into mature breastmilk around three to four days following birth. Colostrum is a thick yellow/orange fluid that is a high-density but low-volume feed present in the first few days following birth, making it the ideal food for newborns. The small volumes facilitate the coordination of sucking, swallowing and breathing at the same time in the first few days of life. Newborns have immature kidneys and are only able to deal with small fluid volumes. Colostrum also has a purgative effect that helps clear the bowel of meconium, which has a high concentration of bile; this in turn reduces the possibility of jaundice.

Colostrum contains higher concentrations of antibodies, and anti-infective properties, such as immunoglobulin A, lysosomes, lactoferrin and white blood cells, than mature milk. It is rich in growth factors and fat-soluble vitamins, particularly vitamin A. It is dynamic, changing nutritional and microbiological content over time which can be affected by diet and mode of birth (Toscano *et al.*, 2017).

Transitional milk

This is the breastmilk produced in the first couple of weeks (lactogenesis II) in which the volume of milk gradually increases, the concentration of immunoglobins decreases and there is an increase in the calorific content, fat and lactose.

Mature milk

The content of mature milk can vary between feeds. At the beginning of the feed, it is high in protein, lactose and water – '*foremilk*', and as the feed progresses, the fat level gradually increases as the milk volume decreases – '*hindmilk*'. This is of particular importance when teaching mothers about the normal pattern of feeding (see Chapter 4). There is a significant increase in the fat content in the morning and early afternoon.

Cregan *et al.* (2002) found the mean milk production for infants up to six months old over a 24-hour period was 809 ± 171 ml, with a range between 549 and 1147 ml, the highest volumes being removed in the morning. Kent (2007) suggested that the maternal energy requirement to produce an average of 759 ml breastmilk per day is 630 kcal.

Constituents of breastmilk

Breastmilk has many properties that meet the individual infant's needs and which, despite improvements in technology, cannot be accurately replicated in artificial milk; breastmilk is often referred to as a 'living fluid'. It is composed of water, fat, protein, carbohydrates, electrolytes, minerals and immunoglobulins.

Fat

This is the main source of energy and provides approximately half of the milk's calories. The lipids are mainly made up of globules of triglycerides, which are easy to digest and make up 98 per cent of the fat content of breastmilk. Breastmilk contains long chain fatty acids, which aid brain and eye development, as well as the nervous and vascular system. However, fat content in breastmilk varies throughout a feed, increasing as the breast is emptied (Czank *et al.*, 2007b). Full breasts are associated with minimum fat content of the milk, while emptier breasts are associated with higher fat content (Kent, 2007; Ballard and Morrow, 2013).

Protein

Protein is essential for growth and development. The ratio of whey and casein proteins changes depending on the stage of lactation from approximately 70/30 or 80/20 in early lactation to 50/50 or 60/40 in more mature breastmilk. Whey remains liquid and contain anti-infective proteins, while casein forms curds and is important to carry calcium and phosphate (Martin *et al.*, 2016; Kim and Yi, 2020). *Lactoferrin* binds iron, promoting easier absorption and preventing the growth of bacteria in the intestine. *Bifidus factor* is also available to promote the growth of *Lactobacillus bifidus* (good bacteria), to inhibit harmful bacteria by increasing the pH of the infant's stool. *Taurine* is also required for the conjugation of bile salts and absorption of fats in the first few days, as well as the myelination of the nervous system.

Probiotics and prebiotics (oligosaccharides)

These interact with intestinal epithelial cells to stimulate the immune system, reduce gut pH to prevent pathogenic bacteria causing infection and increase the numbers of *Bifidus* bacteria on the mucosa (Coppa *et al.*, 2004; Martin *et al.*, 2016).

Carbohydrates

Lactose is the main carbohydrate in breastmilk (98 per cent) and can be quickly broken down into glucose. Lactose is important for brain growth and is found in higher concentration in human milk than in that of other mammals. Lactose is also important in the growth of *L. bifidus*. The amount of lactose in the breastmilk also regulates the volume of milk production through osmosis.

Iron

Healthy term breastfed infants do not require iron supplements before the age of six months (SACN, 2018) because the low levels of iron in breastmilk are bound by lactoferrin, making it more bio-available and thus preventing growth of bacteria in the intestine. Artificial milk has approximately six times more 'free iron', but it is less bio-available, thus promoting growth of bacteria and the risk of infection. Other trace elements are available in lower concentrations than in artificial milk but are considered ideal as they are readily absorbed.

Fat-soluble vitamins

Concentrations of vitamin A and E are adequate for infants. However, vitamins D and K are not always at the desired level. Vitamin D is essential for bone development, but levels are dependent upon the mother's exposure to sunlight. UK Health departments recommend that infants should be given 8.5–10 µg of vitamin D supplements from birth up to one year. In addition, breastfeeding mothers take 10 µg of vitamin D supplements daily (NHS, 2020; SACN, 2016, 2018) (see Chapter 8 for further details).

Vitamin K is required for blood clotting. Colostrum has low levels of vitamin K, and therefore vitamin K is administered routinely to infants at birth. As lactation matures and the infant's gut is colonised with bacteria, vitamin K levels rise.

Electrolytes and minerals

In breastmilk there is a third less electrolyte content and a fifth less sodium, potassium and chloride compared with artificial milk. Calcium, phosphorus and magnesium are present in breastmilk at higher concentrations than in plasma.

Immunoglobins

Immunoglobins are present in breastmilk in three ways and cannot be replicated in formula milk:

• Antibodies from previous maternal infections.
• sIgA (secretory immunoglobin A), which lines the digestive tract.

- The entero-mammary and broncho-mammary pathways (gut-associated lymphatic tissue and bronchus-associated lymphatic tissue). These detect infection in the mother's gastric or respiratory tract and produce antibodies.

White blood cells are present and act as a defensive mechanism to infection; viral fragments prime the baby's immune systems, and anti-inflammatory molecules are thought to protect against necrotising enterocolitis by reducing inflammation in response to pathogens in the gut.

UNICEF UK BFI (2014) produced a useful booklet, *A Guide to Infant Formula for Parents who are Bottle Feeding: The Health Professionals' Guide*, which provides a comprehensive overview of the constituents of breastmilk with references (pp. 17–18).

Volumes of breastmilk

It is important not to try to equate the number and volume of breastfeeds with formula milk. However, many mothers express concern about the amount of milk they are providing for their infants. The following is a guide to average volumes of breastmilk taken during breastfeeding (Kent, 2007).

At birth	Up to 5 ml of breastmilk	First breastfeed
Within 24 hours	7–123 ml/day of breastmilk	3–8 breastfeeds
Between 2 and 6 days	395–868 ml/day of breastmilk	5–10 breastfeeds
At one month	395–868 ml/day of breastmilk	6–18 breastfeeds
At six months	710–803 ml/day of breastmilk	6–18 breastfeeds

It is interesting to note that each breast produces different amounts of milk. In seven of ten mothers, the right breast was found to be more productive (Kent, 2007). Kent (2007) suggests that infants only empty the breast at one or two feeds per day, and, on average, only 67 per cent of the milk available is consumed at an average volume of 76 ml per feed. Since this study, there have been a number of other studies which have found similar results and suggest the lower level of normal milk production by day 11 after birth should be 440 ml (Kent *et al.*, 2016).

Neonatal adaptation to life

Adaptation to extrauterine life

During pregnancy, the mother provides a constant supply of nutrients to the fetus via the placenta. At birth, once the umbilical cord stops pulsating or is cut, there is an abrupt end to the continuous maternal provision of nutrients, and the newborn must adapt to intermittent feeding. The major source of fuel changes from glucose to fat, either from colostrum or neonatal stores.

At birth, infants mobilise stored glucose and fatty acids until a feeding pattern is established. It is normal for plasma glucose levels to decrease within the first two to three hours of life. This coincides with a decreased level of plasma insulin and an increase in plasma triglycerides, fatty acids and glycerol. It is normal for healthy breastfed infants to have lower plasma glucose and higher ketones until lactogenesis II commences than formula-fed infants.

In normal healthy term infants, blood glucose levels can drop to approximately 2.6 mmol/l. Güemes *et al*. (2016) suggest it can vary between 1.4 and 6.2 mmol/l but by 72 hours stabilises to between 3.5–5.5 mmol/l (see local protocol). In response to a low plasma glucose level, serum glucagon levels rise, converting intracellular glycogen stores to glucose (glycogenolysis). The high levels of glucose lead to increased levels of insulin and decreased glucagon levels, but the stores of glycogen decreases rapidly over the first 24 hours after birth. Newborns also have the ability to mobilise alternative fuels through lipolysis and ketogenesis. This is a normal physiological process, and therefore there is no reason to monitor blood glucose levels within the first two to four hours as it will only encourage unnecessary intervention.

Healthy term infants are born with glycogen and fat stores to meet their nutritional needs within the first few days of life while they learn to suckle and feed from the breast. As discussed earlier, colostrum provides all the nutrients required in the first few days of life. The small volume of colostrum, approximately 5 ml at the first feed (Kent, 2007), encourages the coordination of sucking, breathing and swallowing. Due to the small volumes of colostrum, newborn infants will feed regularly, and as a result blood glucose levels are maintained; there is early evacuation of meconium due to the purgative effect of colostrum (reducing the possibility of jaundice); there is promotion of the hormones of lactation, and the mother–baby bond is established.

The mechanisms of suckling

To enable effective removal of breastmilk, human infants are 'hardwired' to suck at birth; however, the birthing environment must support these natural mechanisms. Sucking movements have been observed in utero from 14 weeks, but it is not until 32 weeks' gestation that a fetus or premature infant is able to coordinate the suck and swallow responses and approximately 34–36 weeks' gestation to suck, swallow, breathe and feed at the breast.

Neurobehavioural programme

Nils Bergman (Bergman *et al*., 2019) promoted zero separation of mother and newborn infants, suggesting there is a window of opportunity whereby the infant's innate survival programmes are developed or suppressed. The newborns behaviour is directed by the limbic system via the autonomic nervous system, hormonal system and muscular (somatic) system. Together they achieve the optimum state for current and future health, development and well-being. Furthermore, Bergman and Bergman (2014) suggested separation in the early hours following birth disrupts essential brain development.

Bergman *et al*. (2019) highlighted the importance of the 'first hour' following birth. They identify the mother's smell and skin-to-skin contact as the most important stimuli at birth, as they directly affect emotional memory and fear conditioning. Bergman *et al*. (2019) recommended separation be avoided at this time and that the mother–infant dyad be left undisturbed for a minimum of one hour. This should not be viewed as a one-off process; instead, mother–infant contact should be encouraged as an ongoing process when possible.

Widström *et al*. (2011) suggested that newborn infants should remain in uninterrupted, continuous skin-to skin contact with their mothers in the first hours following birth and that hospital practises should not interfere with this process. They identify nine behavioural stages during the first hour following birth that facilitate and promote breastfeeding and attachment:

1 The birth cry: initial lung expansion
2 Relaxation: no visible movements
3 Awakening: eyes open, small mouth movement
4 Activity: finger and movements, head lifting
5 Resting between stages
6 Crawling: movement towards the breast and nipple
7 Familiarisation: touch, lick, taste the nipple
8 Suckling: self-attachment to the nipple
9 Sleeping

The prone position of skin-to-skin contact allows the infant to move her or his neck and lead with the chin to find the nipple (*rooting response*). When the infant reaches the nipple, it brushes against the philtrum (between nose and upper lip), and the infant opens her or his mouth in a 'wide gape' (*gape response*). The infant takes a mouthful of nipple and surrounding breast tissue and begins to suck. Matthiesen *et al.* (2001) video recorded and observed ten newborn infants in skin-to-skin contact from birth to the first breast-feed; the mothers had not had analgesia. They found that the infants used their hands as well as mouths to stimulate the breasts, resulting in oxytocin release in a coordinated fashion.

Sucking

In a study using ultrasound to observe the movements of the tongue during breastfeeding, Geddes (Geddes, 2007a; Geddes *et al.*, 2021) found that vacuum (negative pressure) played a greater role in the removal of milk than previously thought, suggesting that the creation of negative pressure is an essential component of this process.

Geddes (2007a) described the nipple or areola being drawn into the mouth by negative pressure to the anterior point of the junction of the hard and soft palate. A teat is formed, and the vacuum (–60 mmHg) holds the teat in place. Vacuum occurs as the tongue and jaw move down, drawing milk from the breast. As the tongue rises, the vacuum decreases, reducing milk flow.

At term, the design of the newborn's mouth assists with this action as the tongue is large, filling the mouth alongside the breast. The cheeks also have thick pads of fat and muscle, *buccinators*, which prevent collapse when the tongue depresses during sucking. If the cheeks collapse (appear drawn in), this reduces the negative pressure. The *temporalis* and *masseter* muscles coordinate the symmetrical movement of the jaw during sucking, raising the mandible during the positive pressure phase of the suck and lowering it during the negative pressure phase. The newborn can protect its airway from aspiration because the epiglottis and soft palate touch at rest, diverting the milk to the oesophagus (Watson-Genna and Rabin, 2022).

During attachment to the breast, the lower lip flanges outward on the breast. If the upper lip is also flanged out, this may be a sign of poor attachment. The muscle above the lips, the *orbicularis oris*, contracts to maintain the seal, and the *mentalis muscle* at the lower lip assists feeding by elevating and protruding the lower lip (Watson-Genna and Rabin, 2022).

Swallowing

Coordinated swallowing is evident from 32–34 weeks' gestation. It is triggered by the bolus of milk that accumulates between the palate and the tongue. Watson-Genna and Rabin (2022, pp. 12–13) describe three phases to sucking:

1 *Oral phase*: This involves rooting, attachment and sucking. As the jaw drops, negative pressure is exerted, creating a vacuum to encourage milk to flow from the breast. The tongue forms a trough to channel the milk to the back of the mouth. Milk is delivered onto the tongue.
2 *Pharyngeal phase*: This involves airway protection. Breathing stops, the soft palate rises to close off the nasal cavity, the vocal cords close the trachea and the hyoid bones rise anteriorly, elevating the larynx. As the tongue moves posteriorly, the vacuum reduces and milk flow ceases, the epiglottis moves back and downwards, closing the larynx and diverting the milk bolus to the oesophagus. This is assisted by the contraction of the pharyngeal wall and opening of the oesophageal sphincter.
3 *Oesophageal phase*: The milk bolus passes through the oesophagus aided by peristaltic movement.

Up-and-down jaw movements do not define characteristics of good attachment and swallowing. Geddes (2021) suggested clinical signs of swallowing may include long 'draws' during suckling and audible sounds of swallowing.

Breathing

As breathing must be coordinated with sucking and swallowing, the airway must be protected. An extended neck assists stabilisation of the airway, and in contrast, flexion of the neck increases the risk of collapse of the airway.

Concluding comments

To be able to advise and adequately support mothers with breastfeeding, it is crucial that healthcare professionals keep up to date with research and develop a good understanding of how breastfeeding works to underpin their practice and to be able to effectively pass this information on to mothers in language they understand. The following chapter will explore the essential skills required for practice.

True or false quiz			
		True	*or False*
1	The size of the breast determines milk supply.	☐	☐
2	All mothers produce a similar amount of breastmilk.	☐	☐
3	Lactiferous ducts can be found 5–8 mm from the nipple.	☐	☐
4	Mothers have one milk ejection during a breastfeed.	☐	☐
5	Some breastfed infants may need water between feeds.	☐	☐
6	Colostrum has a purgative effect on the infant bowel.	☐	☐
7	The fat content of breastmilk is higher at the end of the feed.	☐	☐

		True	*or False*
8	The factors present in breastmilk that protect the infant from infection are replicated in formula milk.	☐	☐
9	Prolactin is inhibited until the third stage of labour is complete.	☐	☐
10	A build-up of the feedback inhibitor of lactation will increase milk production.	☐	☐

Further reading

- Geddes, D. (2007a) 'Inside the lactating breast: The latest anatomy research', Journal of Midwifery and Women's Health, 52(6): 556–63.
- Geddes, D., Gridnevza, Z., Perella, S., *et al*. (2021) 25 Years of Research in Human Lactation: From Discovery to Translation, Nutrients, 8(12).
- Watson-Genna, C. (2022) Supporting Sucking Skills in Breastfeeding, Burlington: Jones and Bartlett.

4   Essential skills for practice

- Learning outcomes
- Teaching positioning and attachment
- Assessing a breastfeed
- Expressing breastmilk
- Storage of expressed breastmilk
- Concluding comments
- Quiz
- Resources

Many mothers who stop breastfeeding say they would have liked to have breastfed for longer and would have liked more support and guidance (McAndrew *et al.*, 2012; SG, 2017). This chapter focuses on the essential skills required to effectively support breastfeeding, such as effective positioning and attachment, assessing a breastfeed, hand expression, the use of pumps and storage of milk.

Learning outcomes

By the end of this chapter, you will be able to:

- demonstrate effective positioning and attachment of an infant at the breast;
- observe and assess a complete breastfeed;
- teach a mother how to hand express her breastmilk and safely store it; and
- describe the safe and effective use of breast pumps.

Mapping to UNICEF Baby Friendly Initiative (BFI) Education learning outcomes (2019a)
By the end of the programme, students will:

Theme		Learning outcomes
Theme 1: Understand breastfeeding	1.	Have sufficient knowledge of anatomy of the breast and physiology of lactation to enable them to support mothers to successfully establish and maintain breastfeeding.

DOI: 10.4324/9781003282341-4

Theme		Learning outcomes
Theme 2: Support infant feeding	4.	Be able to apply their knowledge and understanding of the physiology of lactation to support women to get breastfeeding off to a good start.
	5.	Be able to apply their knowledge of physiology and the principle of reciprocity to support mothers to keep their babies close and respond to their cues for feeding, love and comfort.
	6.	Have the knowledge and skills to support mothers and babies to maximise breastmilk and breastfeeding, to continue to breastfeed for as long as they wish and to introduce solid foods at an appropriate time.

Teaching positioning and attachment

Positions for breastfeeding

It is important that breastfeeding mothers understand the need for a comfortable and sustainable position when establishing breastfeeding to avoid poor attachment at the breast that will result in ineffective removal of the milk, pain and trauma. Good positioning is different for each mother as many variables are present, such as the size of the breasts. It is important that the mother adopts a position she can sustain. If she is not comfortable, this may cut the breastfeed short, and the infant will not benefit from the full-fat milk at the end of the feed. It will also encourage a build-up of feedback inhibitor of lactation (FIL) and consequently reduce the milk supply.

Although the mother can adopt different positions, it is important to teach some of the key principles which enable the baby to access the breast using instinctive behaviour; the acronym CHIN is a useful way of teaching these:

Close – The baby is close to her or his mother.
Head free – This allows the baby to tilt his or her head back to allow the chin to lead when attaching to the breast.
In line – The baby's head and neck are in alignment to avoid twisting.
Nose to nipple – This encourages rooting and the tilting of the head backwards to scoop the breast in the mouth.

The infant should be held close and brought to the breast rather than the breast to the infant, as this distorts the shape of the breast. Avoiding holding the back of the infant's head is critical for successful breastfeeding; instead, the infant's neck and shoulders should be supported so that the infant can freely move his or her head to find the correct position to lead with the chin, keep the nose free and open the mouth with a wide gape. It also allows the infant to extend his or her neck and stabilise the airway during the suck–swallow–breathe reflex. In contrast, holding the head pushes the nose, top lip and mouth to the breast, flexing the neck. This causes obstruction of the airway and may block the nose against the breast. It may also encourage the mother to press her breast with her fingers to produce a gap to allow the infant to breathe and, in doing so, prevent milk flow and interfere with attachment. By allowing the infant the freedom to extend the neck, the infant is encouraged to approach the breast chin first to scoop the breast into the mouth and keep the nostrils free. Pushing the head against the breast may also result in breast refusal.

The head and neck should be in a straight line. This enables the infant to open her or his mouth wide, with the tongue on the base of the mouth to scoop up the breast. Avoid twisting of the head and neck as this also helps protect the airway and encourages a successful suck-swallow-breathe reflex.

Aligning the infant's nose to the nipple encourages the infant to tilt his or her head backwards and lead with the chin. In this position, the tongue also remains at the base of the mouth so that the nipple is aimed at the junction of the hard and soft palate. The chin should lead and will indent the breast, the lower lip will flange outwards and the infant will scoop the breast into the mouth (see Figure 4.1).

In the early days of breastfeeding, a mother requires support to find comfortable positions. Advise her to make sure that her clothing is not restricting the feed or that hair or jewellery are not in the way. Many mothers feel thirsty when breastfeeding, so having a drink at hand is a good idea. Usually, mothers can sustain positions in which they feel supported by furniture or pillows. Each mother needs to be assessed individually. Considering pillows to support her back or a footstool may be helpful. If she has a painful perineum, she may need a cushion to sit on. When lying flat, using pillows to support her back or head may make the position more comfortable. It may be useful for mothers of small infants to place them on a pillow on the mother's lap; this depends on the size and shape of the mother's breast because this can be a hindrance to larger infants or mothers with large breasts, causing the infant to assume a twisted position.

Some mothers may need additional help in the early days, particularly if they have not breastfed before. In some hospitals, as many as one in three or four mothers will have had a caesarean section. They need advice on the best positions to avoid having their infants lying on their caesarean section wounds. Mothers of twins need additional help to position the infants. These mothers are at greater risk of shorter duration of breastfeeding (Li *et al.*, 2021) (see Chapter 7 for further discussion).

Some mothers find it helpful to support their breasts, particularly if they are soft or large. This can be done by placing the fingers flat against the ribs, under the breast, with the thumb at a right angle to the fingers. Mothers should be advised to avoid shaping the breast as this may inhibit the flow of breastmilk and potentially cause trauma. As long as these principles are adhered to, the infant can feed in any position in a 360-degree

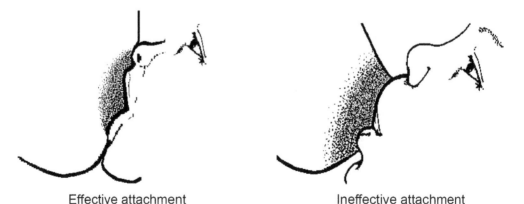

Effective attachment   Ineffective attachment

Figure 4.1 Attachment at the breast

Source: adapted from © UNICEF UK BFI.

circumference of the breast. The following are examples of the more common positions mothers use (Figure 4.2).

- *The cradle position* is the most common position. The mother sits upright, and the infant's neck and shoulders are supported by the mother's forearm or bend in the elbow. Care must be taken not to restrict movement of the head.

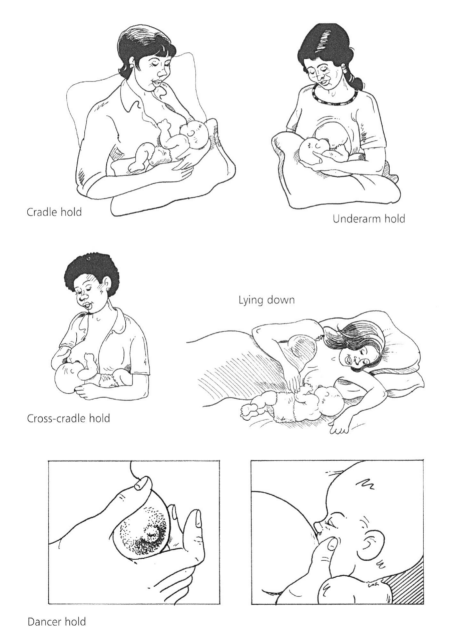

Cradle hold

Underarm hold

Lying down

Cross-cradle hold

Dancer hold

Figure 4.2 Positions for breastfeeding

Source: adapted from © UNICEF UK BFI.

- *The cross-cradle position* is similar except that the baby is supported by the forearm and the neck and shoulders by the mother's hand. It is important that the infant's head is free to move to attain optimal attachment on the breast.
- *The underarm hold* is suitable particularly following a caesarean section to avoid pressure on the wound. Again, the mother sits upright, and she holds the infant to the side, tucking the infant's trunk under her arm with its feet towards her back.
- *Lying down or on the side* is particularly useful if the mother is tired or has a sore perineum. The infant faces the breast, body in alignment, nose to nipple.
- *Straddling* the infant over the mother's legs with the infant sat upright facing the breast is helpful if the infant has congenital hip dislocation.
- *Leaning over the baby* can be useful if the mother has a blocked duct and wants to change the angle of the feed. She places the infant on a secure flat surface, leans over the infant and allows the infant to attach to the breast as usual. This is also useful for mothers with inverted nipples as gravity helps the infant to take a mouthful of breast.

Attachment to the breast

The infant's rooting and suckling reflexes are stimulated by gentle tactile stimulation of the breast. Once the infant has turned towards the nipple and touched it with the lower lip, the reflex to open her or his mouth will be stimulated. The infant will open his or her mouth wide, with the tongue to the base of the mouth. If the mouth is not open wide enough or the tongue is in the roof of the mouth, the infant will be unable to attach effectively to the breast, resulting in 'nipple sucking' (see Figure 4.1) and consequently sore nipples and ineffective milk removal, which may result in insufficient milk supply. Poor attachment can be the precursor to a number of problems discussed in greater detail throughout this book.

The mother must be taught the signs of correct attachment to ensure successful breast-feeding. The steps are:

- Wide-open mouth, tongue on the base of the mouth, scooping a large mouthful of breast.
- Chin indenting the breast.
- Rounded cheeks.
- Rhythmic sucks and the sound of swallowing.
- Seeing milk at the sides of the mouth.
- More areola visible above the top lip than the bottom (although this is difficult for the mother to see in a sitting position).
- The baby finishes the feed and comes off the breast spontaneously.

(See https://www.unicef.org.uk/babyfriendly/baby-friendly-resources/breastfeeding-resources/positioning-and-attachment-video. This video demonstrates how to ensure good positioning and attachment. The site also has other helpful resources for assessment).

Effective attachment is crucial for successful breastfeeding, and midwives, neonatal nurses and health visitors must develop the skills to assess and advise mothers. This is particularly the case in a bottle-feeding culture, where many mothers may not have witnessed successful breastfeeding before, and there is a lack of support from family and friends. However, in a minority of mothers, there may be particular challenges that make it difficult for the infant to attach to the breast. These are explored further in Chapters 6, 7 and 8.

Ineffective attachment

Poor attachment at the breast can lead to a plethora of problems for the mother and infant. For the mother, poor attachment feeding may lead to sore or cracked nipples. If the infant is not properly attached to the breast, this will result in ineffective removal and stasis of breastmilk, leading to engorgement, blocked ducts, mastitis and possible abscess. Because there is ineffective removal of breastmilk, there will be a build-up of the FIL, resulting in a reduced production of breastmilk. The shape of the lactocytes will be distorted, preventing prolactin binding to it and thus slowing down and ultimately preventing further milk production (Czank *et al.*, 2007a).

A poor milk supply leads to the infant's becoming unsatisfied, feeding for a long time or becoming frustrated, showing reluctance to go to the breast and being difficult to settle. The infant is unlikely to empty the breast sufficiently to receive the fattier milk as the breast empties and will become colicky and have explosive, watery and frothy stools. Ultimately, this leads to poor weight gain and failure to thrive. Many mothers perceive this as an inability to produce enough milk to satisfy their infants rather than a problem with technique.

Feeding pattern

At the beginning of a feed before milk ejection, the sucking bursts are rapid, shallow and long with infrequent pauses to swallow. As the feed progresses, the bursts become slower and shorter and the pauses longer until the end of the feed, when sucks become like flutters and the infant releases the breast. The end of the feed is extremely important, and the mother should be advised not to take the infant off the breast prematurely but instead to wait for the infant to release the breast her- or himself because the fat content of the breastmilk is at its highest at that point (Figure 4.3). A sign of good attachment is that the nipple should have maintained a round shape and not be distorted. It is difficult to give a time limit for the length of feeds as this is individual to each infant. At the end of the feed, the infant will become more relaxed and will let go of the breast; the nipple should look round and healthy. In the first few weeks, it is normal for infants to feed approximately 8–12 times a day.

It is important that healthcare professionals recognise factors that affect infants' feeding behaviour. To do this, they must have knowledge and understanding of oral and feeding development in fetuses and newborns (see Chapter 3). Gestational age, illnesses and separation of the mother–infant dyad undoubtedly have an effect and are discussed further in Chapter 8. Maternal factors such as common problems, medication and medical conditions are also considered in Chapters 6 and 7.

Signs of ineffective attachment in the feeding pattern

If an infant continues with rapid sucks and does not demonstrate signs of slow rhythmic sucking, this can be a sign of poor attachment. Other signs are:

- Very long feeds and frequent feeds or very short feeds.
- Colic and frothy, watery stool.
- Breast refusal.

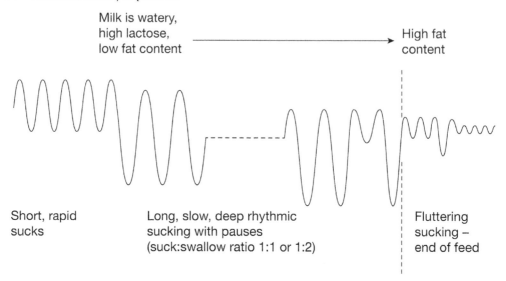

Milk is watery, high lactose, low fat content ————————————→ High fat content

Short, rapid sucks

Long, slow, deep rhythmic sucking with pauses (suck:swallow ratio 1:1 or 1:2)

Fluttering sucking – end of feed

Figure 4.3 The feeding pattern

See Chapter 6 for the management of the consequences of incorrect attachment.

Biological nurturing

Biological nurturing is an approach that offers unrestricted skin-to-skin contact and access to the breast. Colson (2015) states biological nurturing assumptions as:

- Mothers and babies are versatile feeders. There is not one way to breastfeed.
- A baby does not need to be awake to latch on and feed.
- Babies often self-attach; mothers can help them do this.
- Babies often have reflex movements called 'cues' indicating they are ready to feed whilst asleep.
- Looking for baby reflex feeding cues helps mothers to get to know their infants sooner. This increases confidence.
- Crying and hunger cues are late feeding indicators that often make latching difficult.
- The breastfeeding position the baby uses often mimics that in the womb.
- There is no right or wrong breastfeeding position. The right position is the one that works.
- Babies do not always feed for hunger; 'non-nutritive sucking' is hugely beneficial to increase a mother's milk and satisfy her baby's needs.

For further information on biological nurturing, see www.biologicalnurturing.com.

Assessing a breastfeed

Several tools are available to help healthcare professionals to assess breastfeeding technique and to make recommendations for changes to improve breastfeeding outcome. UNICEF UK BFI recommends that a minimum of two breastfeeding assessments be carried out in the first week followed by a plan of care. The BFI has developed checklists to help midwives, neonatal nurses and health visitors as well as mothers recognise that their babies are feeding well, including a bottle-feeding assessment. These can be found at http://www.unicef.org.uk/BabyFriendly/Resources.

Assessing urine and stool

Urine and stool output are fundamental indicators that an infant is feeding well and can be easily recognised by the parents if they are taught to do so. Researchers in California (Nommsen-Rivers *et al.*, 2008) believe that for women to assess their own breastfeeding, they need to be able to assess wet and soiled nappies. They asked 242 mothers to rate the soiled nappies and fullness of their breasts. They found the most effective sign of poor breastfeeding was on day four if there were three or fewer soiled (with stool) nappies. Urine output was less accurate as the mothers were less able to identify this in the nappy. By day three, an infant is expected to produce at least three wet nappies in 24 hours and six or more wet nappies from day five to six (Table 4.1).

The first stool is meconium, which is thick black/green and tarry. This changes over the first few days and is called the 'changing stool' or 'transitional stool'. If an infant is feeding well, the stool can be expected to be yellow by around day five (see Table 4.1).

During the first six weeks, it is expected that a breastfed infant will produce frequent stools (>2 per day). Older infants may have gaps of several days.

Urates and pseudo-menstruation

Urates, which look like orange/pinkish crystals, may be found in the nappies. Parents should be informed that they are salts in the urine and be reassured this is normal for some infants in the first few days. However, urates can be a sign that an infant needs to feed more often or more effectively. This may be a good time to reassess positioning and attachment to prevent any further problems.

Another concern parents may have is pseudo-menstruation. This is a very light bleed from the vagina in some girls and is a result of oestrogen withdrawal. Parents should be reassured that this is normal.

Weighing

All infants are expected to lose weight within the first few days of life, which is thought to be due to normal fluid loss. Infants are born with extra interstitial fluid in their tissues

Table 4.1 Assessing a nappy

Day	Wet nappies per 24 hours	Stools per 24 hours
1–2	One to two or more	One or more (meconium – green/black and sticky)
3–4	Three or more (getting heavier)	Two or more (changing stool)
6	Six or more (heavy)	Three or more (yellow)
Up to six weeks	Six or more (heavy)	At least two (yellow, 'seedy' in appearance)

which needs to be reduced. A normal weight loss is currently considered to be up to 10 per cent of the birth weight, and most infants regain their birth weight within three weeks of birth (NICE, 2018b).

A weight loss over 10 per cent of the birth weight is indicative that the infant is not getting enough milk, and additional support and assessment from a trained professional should be provided. If the birth weight has not been regained by three weeks of age, referral to a paediatrician should be made.

A weight loss of above 12 per cent should be referred to either a general practitioner or paediatrician.

Weight loss must be calculated as a percentage using the following formula:

$$\frac{\text{weight loss (g)}}{\text{birth weight(g)}} \times 100 = \text{weight loss}(\%)$$

Therefore, if the birth weight is 3800 g and the weight loss is 200 g, the weight loss in percentage will be:

$$\frac{200\text{g}}{3800\text{g}} \times 100 = 5.2(\%)$$

In 2009, the World Health Organization (WHO)introduced 0–4 year growth charts for all new births. These charts are based on the growth of breastfed infants. The WHO found that infants worldwide had similar growth patterns and developed the new chart based on data from children who exclusively breastfed for a minimum of four months and partially for one year. The data were collected from infants with no health or environmental factors that may impair the normal growth pattern. Weight should be plotted on the RCPCH UK-WHO growth charts (2013), which include a separate preterm section for infants 32–36 weeks' gestation and a chart for preterm infants born from 23 weeks' gestation. (https://www.rcpch.ac.uk/resources/uk-who-growth-charts-0-4-years).

Materials for training can be downloaded from www.rcpch.ac.uk/growthcharts.

Activity

Read your local guidelines for routine infant weighing policy. The usual pattern for weighing infants initially is at birth (including home births), between days four and six (usually when the blood spot test is done), and around day 10 or 11.

To ensure accurate weight recording, the following guidelines should be followed:

- Use class III electronic or digital scales.
- Weigh babies when they are naked.
- Place scales on a hard surface.
- The infant should be naked in a prone position.
- Weigh before a feed.

- When possible, use the same scales.
- Weighing scales should be serviced annually.

Further information on monitoring weight and faltering growth can be found in Chapter 8.

Expressing breastmilk

Hand expression

Hand expression is a no-cost fundamental technique that should be taught to a mother within 24 hours following birth so she is confident to deal with any issues that may arise, such as supplementing a breastfeed if the infant is ill or unable to breastfeed well at the breast or if they are separated for any reason. It also helps resolve other challenges such as inverted nipples or engorgement. Hand expression provides tactile stimulus, which encourages the hormones of lactation and enables the mother to target specific sites in the breast if she has blocked ducts. If hand expression is the only means of emptying the breast, the mother should be encouraged to express breastmilk at least eight times a day, including during the night when prolactin levels are highest. Hand expression is recommended rather than a breast pump because, in the first few days, colostrum levels are low and may get lost in a breast pump apparatus. Flaherman *et al.* (2012) conducted a randomised control trial of 68 mothers and newborns who were not suckling well at 12–36 hours of age. They found that mothers who hand expressed after birth were more likely to continue breastfeeding at two months than those using mechanical pumping.

Teaching mothers the correct technique for hand expression, as well as a rationale for how breastfeeding works, gives mothers confidence and empowers them to deal with challenges if they arise. Teaching hand expression is best done using a breast model. A 'hands-off' approach should be used unless the mother requests otherwise. NHS UK, UNICEF UK BFI and the Breastfeeding Network have useful videos and resources.

Good breast massage is essential to stimulate milk ejection and should be performed prior to hand expression or when using a pump (Jones and Spencer, 2008). Any of the following techniques can be used; it depends on which the mother finds most comfortable and acceptable:

- Stroke the breast with gentle feather-like movement or gently roll the knuckles from the top of the breast towards the areola.
- Roll the nipple between the thumb and forefinger.
- Stroke under the nipple and areola with the palm of the hand in an upward movement.

Other ways to assist milk ejection are to express near the infant if possible or have a photograph or a piece of the infant's clothing nearby; the smells and sounds of the infant stimulate milk ejection – the let-down (Uvnäs-Moberg and Prime, 2013). Anxiety is a known inhibitor of the let-down reflex; therefore, consideration must be given to the environment, particularly if it is not the mother's own home. In the hospital, a private area should be offered where she knows she will not be interrupted. Physical comfort is also important, so the mother should be reminded to empty her bladder before commencing and ensure she has a comfortable chair, a drink nearby and anything else she may need.

Teaching hand expression

- Wash hands (but not the breast) with soap and water before expressing. Good daily hygiene is sufficient.
- Have a clean container to collect the breastmilk and a towel to place under the breast in case of spillage.
- Encourage the mother to feel gently around the area of the areola, where she will feel a different consistency in the tissue.
- Ask her to place her thumb and first two fingers in a 'C' shape, at 6 and 12 o'clock, approximately 2–3 cm above the nipple (Figure 4.4).
- She should then gently compress the breast and release to express the breastmilk. Some mothers may need to compress the breast and push back to the chest wall. Mothers will find their own rhythm.
- As the drops of breastmilk reduce and stop, she should move her fingers to a different position to drain all the ducts. However, this will not be necessary if the purpose of the expression is just to soften the breast.
- Mothers should be taught to avoid squeezing or sliding their fingers over the skin as this may cause breast tissue damage. They should also avoid pulling on the nipple as this may cause trauma.

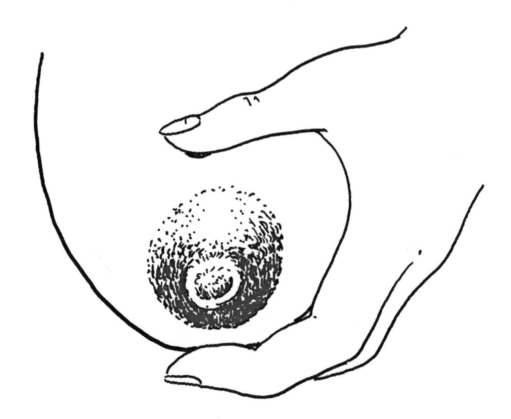

Figure 4.4 Hand expression

It is important to remind mothers that, in the first few days following birth, volumes of colostrum are low and not to expect too much. Once they gain confidence, some mothers may choose to hand express both breasts at the same time. UNICEF UK BFI has a checklist for the assessment of breastmilk expression, which can be found at www.unicef.org. uk (UNICEF UK BFI, 2017b).

Tip

A very rough estimate to guide mothers on how much milk to express per day is 700–900 ml/day (unicef.org.uk).

Breast pumps

Mothers are increasingly using breast pumps as part of their breastfeeding 'toolkit', and it is therefore imperative that healthcare professionals can support and advise them on the benefits and risks of their use and how to use them safely. Mothers of preterm infants use breast pumps to establish and maintain their milk supply. Others use breast pumps to express breastmilk for when they are separated from the infants for an evening out or to return to work. However, if used incorrectly, breast pumps can cause pain, nipple and breast tissue damage, milk contamination and infection (Buckley, 2009). Buckley (2009) described the breast pump as a 'double-edged sword'; on one side, it is invaluable for mothers and infants with breastfeeding problems, but on the other side, there are risks. She questions whether healthcare professionals recommend the use of breast pumps too quickly rather than using clinical observation, teaching the skill of hand expression and providing adequate support and advice.

Electronic breast pumps are composed of a breast shield that sits over the nipple and areola on the breast and the pump, which creates the vacuum to express the milk. They are designed to imitate the infant's suckling, vacuum and sucking rhythm. Two-phase pumps begin with a faster rhythm to initiate the let-down reflex, gradually slowing down as the milk flows. Equipment can be bought or rented. It is helpful if midwives and health visitors can provide a list of local organisations that provide a rental service. Some mothers buy hand pumps, which are cheaper and can be either electronic or manually operated. Suction is created by pumping a handle, but it can be very tiring.

Activity

Write a list of suppliers in your local area where mothers can either buy or rent breast pumps with single-use kits.

If a mother is using a pump to express milk to provide or supplement her infant's nutritional needs, the same instructions regarding how often to do this must be given as for hand expression (see 'Hand expression' earlier).

Not all breast shields fit all mothers, and care must be taken to ensure the shield fits well and will not cause tissue damage. If the procedure is painful, the breast shield could be either too big or too small. Different sizes are available from the manufacturer.

Double pumping (both breasts at the same time) is a good option for mothers who are expressing regularly, as it saves time and increases prolactin levels and therefore milk production. For single pumping, the session should last approximately 15 minutes at each breast, but with double pumping, it should be 10–15 minutes in total.

The mother should:

• Prepare the environment to reduce anxiety levels and aid comfort and have a reminder of the baby if it is not possible to express near the infant, such as a photograph or a blanket.
• Wash hands with soap and water and use a clean pump set (single-person use in hospital).
• Use breast massage to encourage the let-down reflex and continue throughout the procedure.
• Find a comfortable position that can be maintained.
• Support the breast with the fingers flat against the ribs under the breast and with the thumb at a right angle to the fingers.
• Ensure the nipple is placed in the centre of the funnel of the breast shield. The mother should not press the funnel too hard against the breast tissue as this will cause trauma; however, she should make sure it is close enough to maintain the vacuum.
• Start the vacuum on minimum and gradually increase. Kent *et al.* (2008) found in a small study of 23 mothers that expressing breastmilk at a mother's maximum comfortable vacuum enhanced milk flow and yield.
• Do not remove the shield while the vacuum is still on as this will cause nipple or breast trauma.
• Switch breasts as the milk flow starts to slow and swap back.

Kent *et al.* (2008) recommend that mothers use the maximum comfortable vacuum of a breast pump to maximise milk flow rate and yield. At this level, they found there was an average of 4.3 milk ejections in a 15-minute period of expression, yielding 118.5 ml of breastmilk, which is approximately 65 per cent of the available milk.

Mothers should be advised not to reduce the amount of pumping if the milk yield increases beyond what is needed by the infant because if milk is only collected from the first phase of pumping, it will not contain the high fat content of the later milk production. Also, if the intervals between pumping increase, this will lead to a decreased milk production due to the build-up of FIL and reduced prolactin. Instead, the excess could be frozen or offered as donor milk (see Chapter 9 for donor milk guidelines).

Cleaning breast pump equipment

A joint working group of the Healthcare Infection Society and Infection Prevention Society developed best practice guidance for the safe cleaning and decontamination of breast pump kits and other infant feeding items (Price *et al.*, 2016). Key recommendations include:

• Breast pump milk collection kits should not be reused by different mothers unless they have been sterilised in a sterile services department between these different users.

- When used by the same mother, a detergent wash followed by thorough rinsing and drying after each use gives acceptable decontamination for most circumstances, as long as it is performed correctly.
- Additional decontamination precautions to washing, rinsing and drying may be used if indicated by local risk assessments and on advice from the departmental clinicians and infection prevention and control teams. The microbiological quality of the rinse water is an important consideration, particularly for infants on neonatal units.
- If bottle brushes or breast or nipple shields are used, they should be for use by one mother only. Decontamination should be by the processes used for breast pump milk collection kits.
- Dummies (soothers, pacifiers or comforters) needed for non-nutritive sucking by infants on neonatal units should be for single-infant use. Manufacturers should provide these dummies ready to use and individually packaged. They must be discarded at least every 24 hours or immediately if soiled with anything other than the baby's saliva. No attempt should be made to decontaminate the dummies, either before or during use.

Storage of expressed breastmilk

As described in Chapter 3, breastmilk is a 'living fluid' containing antibodies and anti-infective properties such as immunoglobulin A, lysosomes, lactoferrin and white blood cells. Therefore, the recommendations for storage of breastmilk are significantly different from those for formula milk (Table 4.2). All mothers should be advised to wash their hands thoroughly before expressing breastmilk and to wash containers (preferably glass or hard plastic with a lid) with hot soapy water, rinse them and allow them to air dry before use. Containers should be labelled with the date (and name, particularly if storing breastmilk away from the home). To avoid waste, only the required amounts should be stored in each container, for example, 50–100 ml. The containers should have enough space left to allow for the breastmilk to expand when frozen.

However, in the neonatal unit, additional precautions must be taken. Mothers who are hand expressing should use sterile containers to collect breastmilk (such as an enteral syringe or gallipots) and stored with the infant's name, unit number, and the date and time the milk was expressed. Sterile bottles should be used when using a breast pump, which should be labelled with the same information. It is advisable not to overfill the bottles as there could be wastage.

Breastmilk can be transported within 24 hours if in insulated freezer bag or box with freezer packs and fridge temperature maintained. Otherwise it should be used within four hours. Defrosted frozen breastmilk must be used immediately.

Table 4.2 The storage of breastmilk (for term healthy infant)

Storage	Temperature (°C)	Time
Room temperature	19–26	6 hours
Refrigerator	<4	5 days, but if temperature changes, use within 6 hours or discard
Refrigerator	5–10	3 days
Freezer	−18 to 20	Up to 6 months
Ice compartment		2 weeks

Source: BFN (2019a)

Reheating and defrosting breastmilk

Breastmilk should not be warmed using direct heat or a microwave. A microwave does not heat the milk evenly, can cause 'hot spots' in the milk and can destroy some of breastmilk's properties. Breastmilk can be warmed in a container of warm water, or the container can be placed under warm running water for a few minutes. Frozen breastmilk can either be left in the fridge to defrost or placed under cool running water. Once defrosted, it must be used immediately (BFN, 2019a). Mothers sometimes describe a change in appearance of breastmilk when it is stored due to the separation of the casein and whey. Once shaken, this will rectify itself.

Storage of breastmilk in the neonatal unit

In the neonatal unit, breastmilk should be stored in a fridge designated for this purpose only. Temperature recordings should be taken daily and should not exceed 2–4°C. Expressed breastmilk should be used within 48 hours or frozen in a freezer at a temperature of –20°C for a maximum of six months. Always refer to local guidelines.

Concluding comments

To meet the WHO recommendations of exclusive breastfeeding for six months and to continue for two years and beyond, healthcare professionals must develop the knowledge and skills to support, advise and empower breastfeeding mothers. This chapter has covered the basic skills required to do this. Without effective position and attachment, the breasts will not be emptied effectively, leading to a build-up of FIL and a decrease in milk supply. Many mothers state they discontinue breastfeeding because of insufficient milk supply. Poor position and attachment are the main reasons for this problem and the consequential unsettled infant and, in some cases, extreme weight loss and failure to thrive. UNICEF UK BFI recommends that a minimum of two breastfeeding assessments be carried out in the first week followed by a plan of care and that this should include assessment of milk transfer.

Hand expression and the safe storage of breastmilk are also basic skills that healthcare professionals must be able to teach mothers to empower them to solve their own problems should they arise. Good communication skills are crucial in transferring this knowledge in a way mothers can understand and remember; therefore, both verbal and written information should be provided for all mothers.

Quiz

1 Name the principles of good positioning.
2 What position might you recommend for a mother to hold her infant to breast-feed following a caesarean section?
3 Name five signs of effective attachment to the breast.
4 Name three signs of ineffective attachment.
5 When is the fat content of the feed at its highest?

6 When does the BFI recommend all breastfeeding mothers should have a feeding assessment and why?
7 How can you assess adequate milk transfer?
8 If separated from her infant, how many times a day should a mother express breastmilk?
9 Describe the technique of hand expression.
10 Why would you recommend a mother to 'double pump'?

Resources

Positioning and attachment video: Baby Friendly Initiative (unicef.org.uk)

- Breastfeeding Videos: Best Beginnings: bestbeginnings.org.uk/watch-from-bump-to-breastfeeding-online
- Growth chart information: Growth charts (rcpch.ac.uk)
- Suzanne Colson's Biological Nurturing: www.biologicalnurturing.com

5 Good practice to promote, initiate and support breastfeeding

- Learning outcomes
- Building a firm foundation (stage 1)
- An educated workforce (stage 2)
- Parents' experiences (stage 3)
- Concluding comments
- Scenarios
- Quiz
- Further reading and resources

In 2000, Renfrew *et al.* (p. 15) conducted a systematic review of interventions that support or interfere with breastfeeding and identified the following 'key practice areas' that supported breastfeeding, which still resonate today:

- A positive informed attitude to breastfeeding.
- Effective positioning and attachment.
- Pain-free, effective feeding.
- Flexible patterns of feeding.
- No routine use of bottles, teats, dummies and nipple shields.
- Evidence-based practice in maternity units.

The UNICEF UK Baby Friendly Initiative (BFI) best practice standards has been identified as one way to increase breastfeeding rates (Entwistle, 2013; Rollins *et al.*, 2016; WHO/UNICEF, 2021). This chapter focuses on evidence-based good practice to promote and support breastfeeding based on the UNICEF UK BFI standards (2017a), as well as practices that may interfere with successful breastfeeding.

Learning outcomes

By the end of this chapter, you will be able to:

- identify evidence-based practice that will promote, initiate and support breastfeeding;
- avoid practices that interfere with successful breastfeeding; and
- provide individualised education and support to help mothers initiate and maintain lactation.

DOI: 10.4324/9781003282341-5

Mapping to UNICEF UK BFI Education learning outcomes (2019a)
  By the end of the programme, students will:

Theme		*Learning outcomes*
Theme 2: Support infant feeding	4.	Be able to apply their knowledge and understanding of the physiology of lactation to support women to get breastfeeding off to a good start.
	5.	Be able to apply their knowledge of physiology and the principle of reciprocity to support mothers to keep their babies close and respond to their cues for feeding, love and comfort.
	6.	Have the knowledge and skills to support mothers and babies to maximise breastmilk and breastfeeding, to continue to breastfeed for as long as they wish and to introduce solid foods at an appropriate time.
Theme 3: Support close and loving relationships	9.	Develop an understanding of the importance of secure mother-infant attachment and the impact this has on their health and emotional wellbeing.
	10.	Be able to apply their knowledge of attachment theory to promote and encourage close and loving relationships between babies, their mothers and families, irrespective of their feeding method.

Building a firm foundation

Stage 1

- Have written policies and guidelines to support the standards.
- Plan an education programme that will allow staff to implement the standards according to their role.
- Have processes for implementing, auditing and evaluating the standards.
- Ensure there is no promotion of breastmilk substitutes, bottles, teats or dummies in any part of the facility or by any of the staff.

UNICEF BFI (2017a)

Breastfeeding policy

The BFI standards (UNICEF, 2017a) state that healthcare facilities should have a written breastfeeding policy (guideline or protocol) that covers the standards accompanied by a written commitment by relevant managers and adheres to the WHO Code (1981). The policy must demonstrate collaborative working, be routinely communicated to all healthcare staff and all new staff must be orientated to it. During the BFI accreditation process, healthcare facilities are required to demonstrate that all staff involved in providing care for breastfeeding mothers comply with the policy and that a staff education programme is in place.

A named lead for implementation, audit and evaluation is required. It is important that this person has the specific knowledge and skills required as well as dedicated time to perform the role. UNICEF UK BFI have guidelines and tools available at www.unicef.

org.uk/babyfriendly/- resources to monitor and identify when organisations are ready for accreditation.

Avoiding supplements

Breastmilk is the natural food for human infants and provides all the nutritional and immunological requirements to meet the individual needs of healthy term infants until the age of six months and in addition to solid food for two years and beyond (WHO, 2021a). Despite the increase in breastfeeding rates, exclusive breastfeeding until six months continues to be a problem (see Chapter 1). The WHO defines exclusive breast-feeding as when infant 'only receives breastmilk without any additional food or drink, not even water' (2023). The term 'supplementation' can be confusing and often means giving another feed in addition to, or in place of a breastfeed, such as formula or even water. The reasons for giving supplementary feeds include medically indicated reasons, lack of evidence-based practice and parental choice and are discussed further in Chapter 9. Unless medically indicated, supplementing breastfeeds should be avoided because it can increase the risk of allergies and gastrointestinal and respiratory infections and encourage premature cessation of breastfeeding (Renfrew *et al.*, 2012). Giving supplements can have an adverse effect on milk supply because it reduces the number of times the breasts are stimulated through suckling to produce prolactin. The ineffective removal of milk will also lead to a build-up of the FIL and ultimately decrease milk production (Figure 5.1).

The WHO Code (1981) states that mothers should not be given free samples of breast-milk substitutes to take home from hospital because it increases the likelihood that they will bottle feed.

Avoiding teats and dummies (pacifiers)

Nipple confusion can be defined as the interference of artificial nipples such as teats and pacifiers or dummies with the successful initiation of breastfeeding. The use of dummies or pacifiers is common practice in the UK, and the recommendation by UNICEF UK BFI to avoid their use has been a contentious issue among mothers and healthcare professionals. This argument was exacerbated by the inclusion of dummies as a preventative measure against cot death (sudden infant death syndrome [SIDS]) in 2007 by the Foundation for the Study of Infant Deaths (FSID). The FSID suggested that providing a dummy to settle the infant to sleep, even for naps, could prevent cot death. The Lullaby Trust (formerly FSID) updated their guidance in 2022 'Safer Sleep', and there is a section on dummies, stating, 'Some research suggests that using a dummy when putting a baby down to sleep could reduce the risk of SIDS but it is advised to wait until after breastfeeding is established' (https://www.lullabytrust.org.uk/safer-sleep-advice/dummies-and-sids/).

Jaafar *et al.* (2016a) conducted a Cochrane review and found moderate-quality evidence that dummy use in healthy term breastfeeding infants does not reduce the duration of breastfeeding up to four months of age. However, they do caution that there is insufficient information on the potential harms of dummies on infants and mothers. Lubbe and ten Ham-Baloyi (2017) reviewed the literature in this area and suggest dummies could be used in justifiable situations, but guidelines should be available for clinicians. Similarly,

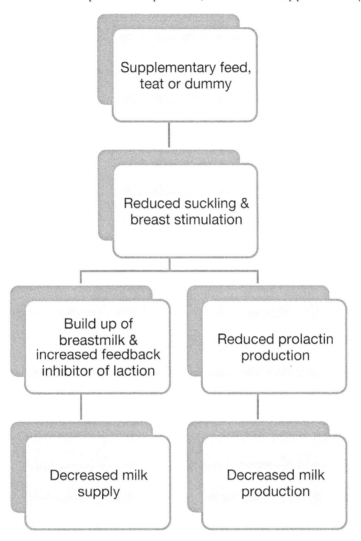

Figure 5.1 The effects of supplementary feeds, teats or dummies

Alm *et al.* (2015) conducted a literature review, finding evidence that breastfeeding and use of dummies reduced the risk of SIDS. They asserted that there was a reluctance to endorse dummy use in case it did have a detrimental effect on breastfeeding, but recent evidence suggests that may not be the case.

To date the main problems identified with introducing teats or dummies appear to exist within the first few weeks following birth, as breastfeeding is becoming established, and are associated with the following problems:

- Altered suck-swallow-breathe cycle, and lower oxygen saturation in preterm infants.
- Reduced number of breastfeeds per day.

- Decrease in milk production due to lack of breast stimulation (see Figure 5.1).
- Early cessation of breastfeeding.
- Increase in tooth decay.
- Increase in ear infections.
- Potential introduction of *Candida albicans* (thrush).

UNICEF UK BFI recommends that when supplementary feeds are necessary, an alternative method of feeding is used, such as cup feeding, to avoid artificial teats; this is discussed further in Chapter 9.

An educated workforce

Stage 2

Educate staff to implement the standards according to their role and the service provided.

UNICEF BFI (2017a)

Healthcare professionals' lack of knowledge and skills to support mothers to breastfeed their infants have been identified as a major contributing factor in low rates of initiation and duration of breastfeeding, leading to inconsistent and inaccurate advice (Renfrew *et al.*, 2005; Balogun *et al.*, 2016; Gavine *et al.*, 2016). It has been suggested that this may be due to a lack of formal education opportunities and 'chaotic' learning environments (Renfrew *et al.*, 2005; McFadden *et al.*, 2007). Robust evidence about healthcare professionals' education in breastfeeding is scarce, so it cannot be assumed that all professionals have the knowledge and skills to provide adequate support and advice for mothers. McAndrew *et al.* (2012) found that three in five mothers said they would have liked to breastfeed for longer. Whilst this was an improvement on the 2005 *Infant Feeding Survey*, most women who had problems were combining breast and formula. The reasons given by those who did stop were insufficient milk, breast refusal or problems with latching on, painful nipples and baby being constantly hungry. This highlights the need for education to be focused on the fundamentals of breastfeeding, communication and problem-solving ability to enhance mothers' confidence but also on the ability teach mothers, particularly where issues can be complex and often contentious and where professionals have their own personal beliefs and attitudes (Gavine *et al.*, 2016).

As part of the BFI accreditation process in stage 2 (UNICEF BFI, 2017a, p. 11), the education staff receive and the knowledge they have to implement the standards is assessed. This includes the skills staff require to support mothers who breastfeed and formula feed ensuring their understanding of the *Code of Marketing of Breastmilk Substitutes*.

There appears to be a consensus that to ensure health professionals provide competent and confident support for mothers who breastfeed their infants, provision of effective education and training is essential in undergraduate programmes as well as continuous professional development (Renfrew *et al.*, 2005; McFadden *et al.*, 2007; Ingram *et al.*, 2011). Several studies have demonstrated that structured evidence-based training programmes for healthcare professionals increase confidence, knowledge and skill. For example, Kronborg *et al.* (2007) suggested that introducing an interactive programme for health visitors improved their knowledge and self-efficacy. Likewise, Ingram *et al.* (2011) found health visitors, nursery nurses and managers reported the three-day BFI course had a positive impact on enthusiasm, confidence and improved consistency when providing advice. These findings are supported by Beake *et al.* (2011), who conducted a systematic review to compare structured and non-structured breastfeeding programmes. Despite overall poor quality of studies, structured programmes were found to have greater influence on initiation and duration of breastfeeding, particularly in areas with low breastfeeding rates.

Whilst the need for continuous professional development and education is evident, employers questioned why midwives and health visitors are exiting their educational programmes without the essential knowledge or skills for practice. In response to this criticism, the UNICEF UK BFI developed the *Best Practice Standards for Higher Education Institutions* in 2002, along with an accreditation procedure which was updated in 2014 and again in 2019 *UNICEF UK Baby Friendly Initiative University Standards* to reflect the new standards (see Appendix 1). In January 2022, 36 per cent of midwifery programmes and 15 per cent of health visiting programmes had full BFI accreditation; in addition, 75 per cent of midwifery programmes and 30 per cent of health visiting programmes are working towards it.

Parents' experiences

Stage 3

Parents' experiences of maternity services

- Support pregnant women to recognise the importance of breastfeeding and early relationships for the health and wellbeing of their baby.
- Support all mothers and babies to initiate a close relationship and feeding soon after birth.
- Enable mothers to get breastfeeding off to a good start.
- Support mothers to make informed decisions regarding the introduction of food or fluids other than breastmilk.
- Support parents to have a close and loving relationship with their baby.

Parents' experiences of neonatal units

- Support parents to have a close and loving relationship with their baby.
- Enable babies to receive breastmilk and to breastfeed when possible.
- Value parents as partners in care.

Parents' experiences of health visiting and public health nursing services

- Support pregnant women to recognise the importance of breastfeeding and early relationships for the health and wellbeing of their baby.
- Enable mothers to continue breastfeeding for as long as they wish.

- Support mothers to make informed decisions regarding the introduction of food or fluids other than breastmilk.
- Support parents to have a close and loving relationship with their baby.

Parents' experiences of children's centres

- Support pregnant women to recognise the importance of early relationships for the health and wellbeing of their baby.
- Protect and support breastfeeding in all areas of the service.
- Support parents to have a close and loving relationship with their baby.

UNICEF BFI (2017a)

Antenatal preparation

The *Infant Feeding Survey 2010* (McAndrew *et al.*, 2012) reported that whilst 96 per cent of UK mothers attended antenatal care, only 38 per cent attended antenatal classes. Similar to Bolling *et al.* (2007), they found attendance at antenatal classes was influenced by the parents' socio-economic background and ethnicity: white mothers were more likely to attend classes (40 per cent) than Asian mothers (25 per cent). For some mothers, becoming pregnant may be the first time they have considered the issue of infant feeding. It may also be the first time they have received any evidence-based information on infant feeding practices. One of the aims of antenatal education is to inform pregnant women about the benefits of breastfeeding to help them be successful and avoid problems.

Advantages of antenatal education are that it:

- provides mothers with knowledge to make informed choices;
- increases confidence;
- increases breastfeeding rates; and
- dispels myths.

UNICEF UK BFI recommends that all mothers have the opportunity for a discussion about feeding their babies and how to recognise and respond to their babies' needs. The focus is now on meaningful conversations as opposed to imparting information; see Chapter 12 for further detail. This can be on a one-to-one basis or as part of an antenatal class. However, a Cochrane review conducted by Lumbiganon *et al.* (2016) was unable to make any recommendations for the content of antenatal breastfeeding education due to methodological limitations of available studies. However, UNICEF UK BFI has a series of resources on its website to support meaningful conversations in pregnancy. The key points they recommend for discussion in the antenatal period are:

- *Encourage parents to connect with their baby:* take time out to connect: talk to baby, notice and respond to movements.
- *Skin contact:* the value of skin contact, what this means for mother and baby, sharing the value of skin contact.
- *Respond to the baby's needs:* how closeness, comfort and love can help baby's brain develop; responsive feeding.
- *Feeding:* The value of breastfeeding as protection, comfort and food; how to get off to a good start.

Some clinicians recommend antenatal expression of breastmilk to mothers who are at risk of preterm birth or whose infants are high risk and may have difficulty breastfeeding initially (see Chapters 7 and 8). The intention is that the infant can receive expressed colostrum if supplementation is required instead of formula milk. This process can commence at around 36 weeks of pregnancy but should be stopped if any uterine contractions or tightening are felt and is contraindicated if there is a history of threatened or premature labour, multiple pregnancy, cervical incompetence or cervical suture in situ. The procedure is the same as for the expression of milk. However, colostrum will only be expressed in small amounts and should be collected in small sterile syringes or other suitable receptacles so that none of it is wasted. If colostrum is expressed more than once a day, a new receptacle should be used each time. The colostrum should be frozen at −18°C and labelled appropriately. If the mother is bringing it into hospital, it will require a name, date and identifying number (see Chapter 4).

Skin-to-skin contact

Despite differences of the timing of the first breastfeed in different cultures, it is strongly recommended that skin-to-skin contact should take place as soon as possible following birth. The dried infant is laid on the mother's bare chest after birth, and both are covered with a blanket to keep them warm. Unhurried skin-to-skin contact should not be interrupted to provide routine care such as weighing the infant or bathing. UNICEF UK BFI recommends that all mothers should have skin-to-skin contact with their baby after birth, at least until the first feed and for as long as they wish, and be encouraged to offer the first feed in skin contact when the baby shows signs of readiness to feed. Infants of these mothers should be kept in skin-to-skin contact for as long as possible.

There was a significant increase in skin-to-skin contact reported in the *Infant Feeding Survey 2012* (McAndrew et al., 2012) compared with 2005 (Bolling et al., 2007): 81 per cent within the first hour, increasing to 88 per cent within 24 hours. The survey also identified a link between increased breastfeeding initiation with babies who had skin-to-skin contact.

When a mother and infant are separated for clinical reasons, skin-to-skin contact should commence as soon as the mother and infant are able to do so. During unrestricted skin-to-skin in the first hour following birth, oxytocin levels are high (Nissen et al., 1996), which, as well as encouraging the let-down reflex, facilitates instinctive breastfeeding behaviour in both the mother and the infant or, as described by Nils Bergman (2019), the neurobehavioural programme (Figure 5.2). Moore et al. (2016) conducted a systematic review of 38 studies, including 3,472 mother–infant dyads. They found evidence to support immediate or early skin-to-skin contact in the promotion of breastfeeding and should be normal practice for healthy term infants, including following caesarean section.

If infants are separated from their mothers, they display signs of 'hyper-arousal response', in which the heart rate, respiratory rate and blood pressure increase (Bergman, 2019), even if this is in a cot in the same room. They cry much more than usual, in short pulses, which is possibly a distress call for the mother as exhibited in other mammals and which may impair lung and cardiac function, increase intracranial pressure and initiate stress reactions that can have long-term negative effects (see Chapter 2).

Skin-to skin contact can be initiated for infants of any age. It helps to calm the infant and can also help when there are problems with attachment or other common problems (Svensson et al., 2013) (see Chapter 6).

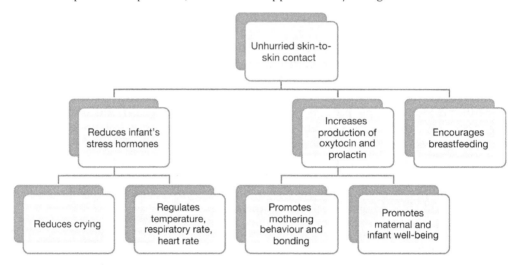

Figure 5.2 The benefits of skin-to-skin contact

Kangaroo care

To improve outcomes, pre-term or low birth weight infants should be supported to have kangaroo care, including skin-to-skin contact, immediately after birth rather than waiting for the infant to be stabilised in an incubator (WHO, 2021b). It promotes physiological and emotional outcomes such as cardiorespiratory stability, thermoregulation, sleep, and effective procedural pain relief. In addition, it reduces cortisol levels and infection and increases oxytocin levels (Campbell-Yeo *et al.*, 2015). In turn this promotes growth and brain development. Campbell-Yeo *et al.* (2015) found evidence to support the influence of kangaroo care on breastmilk volume, initiation of earlier breastfeeding and longer duration as well as increased attachment behaviours. UNICEF UK BFI provide a practical skills review form for kangaroo care which is available on their website. This includes guidance on transferring an infant to the parent or incubator safely.

Responsive feeding

Restricting infant feeds was introduced in the early twentieth century in an attempt to make breastfeeding more scientific. It was thought that an infant's stomach needed three to four hours to empty and that prolonged feeding could cause problems such as diarrhoea and vomiting. It is now widely accepted that restricting breastfeeds can lead to an insufficient milk supply, failure to thrive and early cessation of breastfeeding. Many health professionals refer to 'baby-led' or 'demand feeding', but UNICEF UK BFI (2016b, p. 1) does not believe this clearly explains breastfeeding and recommend using the term *responsive feeding*, which

'. . . involves a mother responding to her baby's cues, as well as her own desire to feed her baby. Crucially, feeding responsively recognises that feeds are not just for nutrition, but also for love, comfort and reassurance between baby and mother'.

Responsive feeding acknowledges the synchronous relationship between mother and infant, recognising that breastfeeding is a reciprocal relationship between mother and infant that will enhance growth, development and emotional attachment.

Readiness to feed is an important skill for mothers to learn. Entwistle (2013, p. 74) suggests an infant who is ready to feed is:

- visually attentive to their mother – eyes opening, eye contact and gazing; smiling (if old enough);
- making vocal sounds directed towards their mother (no crying);
- showing relaxed, quiet movements, moulding to the mother's body; and
- displaying feeding cues such as stretching the arms and legs, murmuring or making rooting or sucking movements.

It is important a mother spend the first few weeks bonding with her infant, learning the infant's feeding cues and behaviour. Crying is considered a late sign of hunger, and it is important to teach the mother earlier signs that her infant needs to breastfeed (Watson and McGuire, 2016).

There are situations that can interfere with this relationship such as use of dummies, separation and a sleepy or sick infant when regular feeding is required as a temporary solution. If there is concern in the early days after birth about the length of time between feeds, the mother may need to wake the infant up and encourage her or him to feed to establish or maintain lactation to avoid a build-up of the feedback inhibitor of lactation, which will cause inhibition of milk production. It is also important for the mother to avoid her breasts becoming too full and uncomfortable, leading to engorgement, blocked ducts or mastitis.

Parents are often concerned about time limits and should be advised that every infant's requirements will be different. However, on average, infants should breastfeed about eight times in a 24-hour period. They may find at some times in the day that the infant will cluster feed and then go for longer periods at another time. There may be medical requirements when the infant's condition does not allow responsive feeding and the infant needs to feed frequently and regularly. However, as soon as possible, responsive feeding should be encouraged.

While in hospital, it is important that hospital routines and procedures do not interfere with responsive feeding (such as mealtimes, examination, ward rounds). Also, in the home, visitors should not disrupt this process. Some mothers find visitors keen to come and help with the infant; however, it would be more beneficial if they helped with domestic chores and allowed the mother and infant to be together.

The benefits of responsive feeding include:

- maintenance of an adequate milk supply;
- less infant weight loss in the immediate postpartum period;
- increased duration of breastfeeding;
- prevention of engorgement, blocked ducts and mastitis;
- reduction in hyperbilirubinaemia (elevation of bilirubin levels causing jaundice);
- a comforted and calm infant; and
- promotion of a close and loving relationship.

Although there is a lack of supporting evidence, UNICEF UK BFI (2019b) recommends mothers who formula feed to be encouraged to feed responsively and be offered support and advised to:

- respond to cues that the baby is hungry;
- invite the baby to draw the teat rather than forcing the teat into the mouth;
- pace the feed so that the baby is not forced to feed more than they want to; and
- recognise their baby's cues that they have had enough milk.

Rooming-in

In the past, most hospitals practised 'nursery care' for infants. The intention was often altruistic, but it had negative consequences for breastfeeding. Nursery care was justified by midwives, who said they were taking the infant away to let the mother rest; however, evidence suggests that mothers actually sleep better when their infants are near due to the oxytocin release (Ball, 2003; Taylor *et al.*, 2015). Separated infants were also at risk of receiving supplementary feeds and dummies. This practice also increased the risk of infection and deprived the mother–infant dyad of the opportunity to interact and develop innate feeding behaviour, maternal feelings and confidence. In contrast, 'rooming-in', or keeping the mother and infant together in the same room, enables the mother to get to know her infant, learn the feeding cues and gain confidence in handling the infant and is a key clinical practice in the 'Steps to Successful Breastfeeding' (step 7). It facilitates unrestricted feeds, which in turn stimulates production of prolactin and empties the breasts regularly. If the mother learns her infant's feeding cues, she can react quickly and breastfeed the infant before he or she becomes too distressed and more difficult to attach to the breast. However, a Cochrane review by Jaafar *et al.* (2016b), which explored the influence of rooming-in versus separate care for infants for increasing the duration of breastfeeding, was inconclusive due to low-quality evidence.

Bed-sharing and co-sleeping

Current advice recommends that the safest place for infants to sleep is in their own cot in the same room as the parents (Lullaby Trust, 2022). Bed-sharing is a contentious issue and often places the promotion of breastfeeding and the prevention of SIDS in conflict. An example of this was the inaccurate media reports on the case-control study conducted in 2009 by Blair *et al.* The media claimed bed-sharing for breastfeeding was contraindicated. The aim of the study had been to ascertain the major risk factors associated with SIDS in 0–2-year-olds. It was conducted over a four-year period in the southwest of England and concluded that many of the infants with SIDS had co-slept in a hazardous environment and that the major influences were parental use of alcohol or drugs prior to co-sleeping or sleeping on the sofa. They suggested that these factors could be addressed by educating parents not to fall asleep with the infant on the sofa and not to co-sleep if they had taken drugs or alcohol.

Helen Ball is a well-known anthropologist who has done a large amount of research into bed-sharing and co-sleeping. She states (Ball, 2009) that anthropologists consider mother–infant sleep as normal for humans and recent research confirms that bed-sharing is common practice. Ball (2002, 2003) conducted a study with 253 families in the northwest of England and reported that 47 per cent slept in the same bed as their one-month-old infants, but this figure dropped to 29 per cent when the infants were three months old. These findings were supported by the *Infant Feeding Survey 2005* (Bolling *et al.*, 2007). Ball (2003) suggested that mothers who share a bed with their infants in the first month are twice as likely to be breastfeeding at four months of age. In 2006, Ball *et al.* conducted a randomised trial of infant sleep location on the postnatal ward. They videoed mother–infant dyads in different locations: (1) the infant in a normal cot by the bed, (2) the infant in a side cot attached to the bed and (3) with the infant in the bed with cot sides. They observed that infants in the side cot or in bed attempted to and successfully breastfed more frequently than those in the standard cot by the bed. The ability to root and suckle was hampered for infants in standard cots, and the mothers were unable to see the feeding cues readily, or their responses were hindered by not being able to access the cot easily and sometimes requiring assistance.

Ball *et al.* (2006) also observed differences in sleep positions between breastfeeding mothers and formula-feeding mothers. Breastfeeding mothers adopted a protective position more often than formula-feeding mothers. They slept facing the infant, on their side with their legs curled under the infant's feet, protecting the infant from some of the risks. The infant's position was level to the breast within the space created by the mother. Formula-feeding mothers spent more time asleep turned away from their infants.

Again in 2016, Ball *et al.*, conducted a randomised trial of 870 women and found women with a strong motivation to breastfeed frequently bed-shared, highlighting the need to provide women with accurate information on how to do this safely.

As discussed in Chapter 2, it is important that mothers are able to respond early to feeding cues, particularly in the first few days, to ensure adequate production of prolactin to prime the lactocytes, to initiate and maintain lactation (lactogenesis II). Night-time feeds are particularly important as greater amounts of prolactin are released.

Key fact

Prolactin levels peak at night (circadian rhythm); therefore, night feeds must be encouraged to promote milk production.

The benefits of sharing a bed are well documented in terms of physical and psychological development and include:

- regulation of breathing, heart rate and thermoregulation;
- improvement of breastfeeding initiation and duration by increasing the frequency of breastfeeds during the night when prolactin levels peak;
- enabling the mother to respond quickly to infant feeding cues;
- reduction in the incidence of SIDS;
- reduction in the incidence of neglect; and
- an increased feeling of closeness and bonding.

However, safety is paramount, and parents must be given information about risk factors associated with bed-sharing and SIDS and how to reduce the risk of accidents or overheating. The Lullaby Trust updated their guidance for co-sleeping 2022 (see lullabytrust.

org.uk for resources), supported by UNICEF UK BFI. It includes the following advice for parents:

- The safest place for your baby to sleep is in a cot by the side of your bed.
- *Never* lie with or co-sleep on the sofa or in an armchair.
- *Do not sleep with the baby if:*
  - You or your partner smoke.
  - You or your partner have taken alcohol or drugs (legal or illegal) are ill or unusually tired or if the infant is unwell and has a high temperature.
  - Your baby was born prematurely (before 37 weeks of pregnancy) or weighed under 2.5 kg when they were born.

In addition to reduce the risk of sudden infant death parents should be advised:

- to put the baby down on their back to sleep, never front or side.
- to place the cot beside the parent's bed for at least the first 6 months.
- to make sure the mattress is firm and flat – no waterbeds or sagging mattresses.
- to not overdress the baby.
- to ensure the room isn't too hot; 16–18°C is ideal.
- to ensure that the room in which the baby sleeps is smoke-free;
- to ensure the partner knows when the infant is taken into bed.

  - to keep pillows and adult bedding away from the baby or any other items that cover their head or cause them to overheat.
  - not to bring other children or pets into bed.
  - to make sure the baby cannot get trapped or wedged between the bed and the wall, or fall out of bed.
  - to never leave the baby unattended in a bed.

It is not safe to bed-share in early months if the baby was born very small or premature.

Teaching a mother to maintain lactation

Many mothers, particularly if they have not breastfed before, need to be shown how to breastfeed and maintain their lactation if separated from their infant. This may include psychological support as well as practical information about technique, such as position and attachment, hand expression and recognising effective milk transfer (see Chapter 4). If the mother and infant are to be separated, it is essential that the mother is taught about hand expression to establish or maintain lactogenesis. This is discussed further in Chapter 4.

Inclusive support for trans and non-binary people

The *Improving Trans Experiences of Maternity Services (ITEMS) project* (LGBT Foundation, 2022) highlights the varied experiences, insights and needs of trans men and non-binary people who have accessed perinatal services. They found many examples of inequalities, discrimination and poor outcomes, most notably those trans men and non-binary respondents who were people of colour. In addition, they also found examples of innovation and a pro-active approach to gender inclusion. However, the study found that fewer than half the trans and non-binary respondents felt their decisions around feeding their babies were always respected by midwives. Not being supported with dignity and respect were highlighted as key barriers to trans and non-binary people accessing services. The report makes the following recommendations to provide an inclusive service and improve their experiences:

1 Targeted information about choices of infant feeding.
2 Inclusive language: Some trans and non-binary people may use the term 'chest feeding or 'body feeding' rather than breastfeeding. Ask about language and how they describe their bodies.
3 Pro-active inclusion: Have visible signs of inclusion such as posters; opportunity to receive feedback on care and co-producing service with local trans and non-binary communities, organisations and groups.
4 Personalised care tailored to address the persons specific needs.
5 Trauma-informed care: Trans and non-binary people are more likely to have experienced trauma than cisgender people, and therefore continuity of care is key to develop a relationship to ensure the persons needs are met, increase satisfaction and improve care and outcomes.
6 Training to deliver gender-inclusive care.
7 Upgrade information technology systems to avoid misgendering people.
8 Demographic monitoring by inclusive gender and trans status questions on evaluation or surveys to benchmark and monitor experiences and outcomes of trans and non-binary people.

Support groups

It is important that breastfeeding mothers do not feel isolated when they leave the hospital, and in recent years, a number of initiatives have been developed to provide support in the community; however, many still require evaluation. It is therefore important to provide mothers with information about the types of support they can access and how to do this. This can be done in the form of a list of contact telephone numbers or websites for midwives, health visitors, support groups (lay and professionals), peer supporters and counsellors. Sources of community support are further explored in Chapter 11.

Concluding comments

The UNICEF UK BFI standards are a good point of reference to identify practices that either support or interfere with successful breastfeeding and have been shown to improve breastfeeding rates (Renfrew *et al.*, 2012; Entwistle, 2013). However, it has to be acknowledged that a great deal more robust research is required to support many areas of practice. Mothers need to be empowered with the correct 'toolkit' from the births of their infants to give them confidence to breastfeed for as long as they choose to, which includes practical skills as well as evidence-based information.

Practice should be developed to meet the needs of the mother and infant rather than organisational processes. It is crucial that there is a health board or authority strategy and policy that has commitment from the executive team and managers and that all relevant healthcare professionals receive adequate training, preferably in the pre-registration programme but also as part of their continuous professional development. By doing this, healthcare professionals will be able to provide consistent and accurate information for mothers and infants in their care. Using the UNICEF UK BFI Standards this chapter has explored how this can be achieved and potential problems avoided. The following chapter explores more specific problems individual mothers may encounter and how they can be resolved. Parents' experiences of neonatal units are discussed in Chapter 8, and health visiting and public health services is discussed in Chapter 11.

Scenarios

1 Jane is 42 years old and gave birth to her baby 11 days ago. Her baby has lost 10 per cent of his birth weight. Her life is hectic, and her other children are four years and 18 months old. The baby is described as a 'crying, fretful baby', and you have implemented good practice for improving weight gain, effective positioning and attachment, and hand expressing. Jane asks you about skin-to-skin contact and guidance on safe bed-sharing:

   • How would you advise Jane?

2 Sharmila is a 22-year-old primigravida who has had a rotational forceps delivery of a 4.5-kg male infant. There was a long labour with an active pushing stage of about two hours. Sharmila is exhausted, and the baby is feeding frequently. She asks if should give the baby a dummy or a bottle so she can get some sleep.

   • What would you say to Sharmila?
   • What can you do to help her?

Quiz

1 Give three reasons why a normal healthy term baby may not feed regularly within the first 24–48 hours.
2 Name four benefits of skin-to-skin contact.
3 List the ways parents can reduce the risk of overheating and accidents if they choose to bed-share.
4 Why is 'rooming-in' recommended?
5 What are the advantages of having a breastfeeding policy for mothers?
6 How can you inform mothers about the breastfeeding policy in your area of practice?
7 What advice would you give a mother who suggests she is going to give her baby a dummy?
8 How would you explain what is meant by responsive feeding?
9 Why should supplementary feeds not be given to breastfeeding infants?
10 Describe the infant feeding cues you should teach mothers to look out for.

Further reading and resources

- Entwistle, F.M. (2013) *The Evidence and Rationale for the UNICEF UK Baby Friendly Initiative Standards*. UNICEF UK. London.

- Renfrew, M., Pokhrel, S. and Quigley, M., *et al.* (2012) *Preventing Disease and Saving Resources: The Potential Contribution of Increasing Breastfeeding Rates in the UK*. London: UNICEF UK.

- Breastfeeding Resources
  www.unicef.org.uk/babyfriendly/baby-friendly-resources/

- From bump to breastfeeding
  www.bestbeginnings.org.uk/from-bump-to-breastfeeding

- Lullaby Trust
  www.lullabytrust.org.uk/safer-sleep-advice/

6 Management of common problems

- Learning outcomes
- Breastfeeding assessment
- Breast refusal
- The reluctant feeder or 'sleepy' infant
- Nipple pain or trauma
- White spot
- Insufficient milk supply
- Inverted nipples
- Breast engorgement
- Blocked ducts
- Mastitis
- Abscesses
- Thrush or *Candida albicans*
- Concluding comments
- Scenarios
- Resources

Many mothers experience common complications of breastfeeding and require skilled support and advice to ensure that lactation continues. McAndrew *et al.* (2012) asked mothers who stopped breastfeeding within the first two weeks why they had done so. The most common reasons were:

- The infant rejecting the breast or not sucking (33 per cent).
- Painful breasts or nipples (22 per cent).
- A perception of insufficient milk (17 per cent).

They also reported that the majority of mothers who stopped breastfeeding within the first two weeks would have liked to have continued and believed the following factors would have helped:

- More support and guidance from hospital staff, midwives and family (23 per cent).
- The infant latching on the breast easier (19 per cent).
- Less pain (14 per cent).

DOI: 10.4324/9781003282341-6

Following on from the essential skills required to support breastfeeding mothers in Chapter 4 and how to promote good practice to support and protect breastfeeding in Chapter 5, this chapter addresses the knowledge and skills required to support mothers with some of the common problems they may experience. It builds on the skills of how to observe effective milk transfer discussed in Chapter 4, beginning with the fundamental skill of undertaking a detailed breastfeeding assessment to identify the root of the problem so that it may be corrected. However, it must be remembered that each mother is an individual, and the management must be skilfully tailored to meet her needs and those of the infant.

Learning outcomes

By the end of this chapter, you will be able to:

- take an accurate breastfeeding assessment;
- identify the common complications of breastfeeding;
- diagnose the common complications of breastfeeding;
- teach a mother how to avoid the common complications of breastfeeding; and
- describe safe and effective techniques and treatments for the common complications of breastfeeding.

Mapping to UNICEF UK Baby Friendly Initiative (BFI) Education learning outcomes (2019a)

By the end of the programme, students will:

Theme		Learning outcomes
Theme 2: Enabling mothers to breastfeed	6.	Have the knowledge and skills to support mothers and babies to maximise breastmilk and breastfeeding, to continue to breastfeed for as long as they wish and to introduce solid foods at an appropriate time.
Theme 4: Managing the challenges	11.	Be able to apply their knowledge of the physiology of lactation and infant feeding to support effective management of challenges which may arise at any time during breastfeeding.

Breastfeeding assessment

It is acknowledged that problems with breastfeeding can be the result of psychosocial and physical issues, as well as hospital practices, poor advice and a lack of support from healthcare professionals. Therefore, making an accurate breastfeeding assessment is essential to get to the root of the problem and to be able to make an accurate diagnosis. UNICEF UK BFI has developed a range of breastfeeding assessment tools for maternity, health vising, neonatal and for the mother herself, available on the website. They comprise a series of questions to explore the possible situations that may interfere with successful breastfeeding, so that an appropriate and individualised plan of care can be developed. It includes questions on the following areas:

1 Infant's feeding pattern
2 Infant's nappies: frequency and output
3 Breast assessment

The neonatal assessment tool includes an assessment score to determine tube top ups. Good communication skills are key to this process as discussed in Chapter 12.

Key fact

For all breastfeeding problems:

1 Take a history.
2 Observe a complete breastfeed for effective milk transfer:

- Correct position and attachment.
- Including sucking pattern.

3 Observe for breast or nipple anomalies.
4 Assess the infant's mouth for tongue-tie or any other anomaly.
5 Encourage skin-to-skin contact.
6 Use positive language to promote confidence.
7 Produce a care plan to avoid conflicting advice.

Breast refusal

McAndrew *et al.* (2012) found breast refusal to be the most common reason for mothers stopping breastfeeding in the first two weeks. It can be very distressing for mothers and undermine their confidence in their ability to breastfeed. Many mothers report feeling that they take it personally and think the infant may not like them. Infants who refuse to breastfeed may exhibit the following signs:

- Arching of the back.
- Stiffening of the body when approaching the breast.
- Pushing the breast away with arms and legs.
- Crying.
- Extending and turning the head away from the breast.

Breast refusal is commonly associated with an unpleasant event involving breastfeeding, such as someone pushing the head to the breast to encourage feeding. Some mothers report the infant biting them and their startled reaction leading to breast refusal. Other causes may be due to smell, such as changed perfume, washing powder or soap, the taste of the milk due to a change in diet or medication or sometimes the onset of menstruation. There may also be issues with the infant, such as teething, ear or nasal obstruction, thrush or other infection.

Practice recommendations: breast refusal

When there is breast refusal, it is important not to further exacerbate the problem. The aim is to create a relaxed mother–infant dyad by encouraging a calm and relaxing environment.

- Maximise skin-to-skin opportunities, not only at feeding times, and recommend co-bathing.
- Closely observe for feeding cues and initiate a breastfeed before the infant cries.
- If the infant protests (arching of back, pulling away, crying), discontinue the feeding attempt and calm down the infant. Try again once the infant is calm and displaying feeding cues. There is no point in attempting to put the infant to the breast if he or she is distressed.
- If the infant does not breastfeed, express breastmilk and give this via a cup or syringe but try to put the infant to the breast at each feed attempt as described earlier.
- Breastfeed in a relaxed and quiet environment with no interruptions.
- Advice between professionals must be consistent and therefore a care plan is advisable.

Other issues must be excluded, such as birth injury resulting in pain or intracranial haemorrhage, oral aversion following suction at birth or other stimulation, hyperlactation or over-active let-down reflex, insufficient milk supply, nipple–teat confusion and maternal drug abuse or developing illness.

The reluctant feeder or 'sleepy' infant

In the first couple of days following birth infants may feed infrequently, appear sleepy and may not demonstrate feeding cues. Sometimes even if the infant does latch on to the breast, she or he may only take a few sucks and fall asleep. This can be a very frustrating problem for mothers and midwives; however, it must be remembered that normal healthy term infants are not at risk because they are able to mobilise glycogen and ketones for energy. Despite this, it is important for the mother to encourage the infant to breastfeed to promote the production of prolactin. If the infant does not suckle, the mother should hand express at regular intervals. Some of the reasons for a sleepy infant are:

- maternal analgesia in childbirth;
- birth complications that lead to increased levels of endorphins;
- congenital anomalies or illness;
- birth trauma;
- operative delivery;
- hyperbilirubinaemia (jaundice) and phototherapy; and
- prematurity.

Nipple pain or trauma

Painful nipples are one of the most common reasons for mothers seeking help and support or stopping breastfeeding. Nipples may feel sensitive and tender in the early days of breastfeeding but should not be painful. Painful nipples may be associated with sore or cracked nipples, which may have a fissure, blisters and bleeding. If the mother complains of pain in the first few days, it is likely a problem with positioning and attachment. However, pain can also be a symptom of thrush and other problems, which should be ruled out (these conditions are discussed later in this chapter). An open wound in the nipple is also a portal of entry for infection. Other reasons for nipple pain could be Raynaud's disease, eczema, dermatitis or impetigo (Kent *et al.*, 2015).

Raynaud's disease is caused by the short-term but exaggerated vasoconstriction of blood vessels, usually in the extremities such as fingers and toes, leading to hypoxia of the tissue. Raynaud's disease can also be found in the nipple and is a treatable condition, but it is often mistaken for thrush because of the severe pain (Anderson *et al.*, 2004; Barrett *et al.*, 2013). It is associated with cold temperatures and causes blanching of the nipple and sometimes cyanosis or erythema (redness of the skin). Anderson *et al.* (2004) recommended that diagnosis is made when biphasic (cyanosis and erythema) or triphasic (pallor, cyanosis, erythema) colour changes of the nipple are noted. Mothers with this condition may also have experienced these symptoms during pregnancy and when not breastfeeding. Treatment includes avoiding cold temperatures and substances that cause vasoconstriction, such as nicotine and caffeine. However, because the pain is so severe, mothers may need pharmacological intervention, such as nifedipine, which causes vasodilation (Anderson *et al.*, 2004; Barrett *et al.*, 2013).

Practice recommendations: sleepy infant

Mothers can become very upset and express concerns about their ability to breast-feed, so it is extremely important to reassure a mother and teach her techniques that will encourage the infant to feed and encourage milk production. The midwife should regularly assess the feeds and observe the infant to exclude any signs of illness.

- Encourage undisturbed skin-to-skin contact.
- Encourage uninterrupted access to the breast.
- Attempt to put the infant regularly to the breast followed by hand expression of breastmilk, which can then be given to the infant by cup or syringe.
- Reinforce how to recognise feeding cues.
- Ensure the infant is not too hot or cold when feeding.
- If required, use breast compression to encourage the flow of milk. Place the thumb on the upper side of the breast and the other fingers underneath the breast close to the chest wall. Squeeze, hold and release to increase the internal pressure in the breast to release milk.
- 'Switch' feeding may keep the infant awake (changing from one breast to the other several times during a feed).

This problem usually resolves itself within 36–48 hours, when infants will normally breastfeed 8–12 times a day. If the infant is still sleepy, referral to a paediatrician will be required to exclude underlying illness.

Nipple pain can be very distressing for mothers, and the resulting anxiety may inhibit the let-down reflex. It may also lead to reduced frequency and length of breastfeeds or exclusivity of one side, resulting in ineffective removal of breastmilk or even discontinuation of breastfeeding. The aim of treatment is to alleviate the pain while maintaining lactation. Treatment can be difficult because of repeated trauma and potential infection. Therefore, nipples should be assessed and treatment determined on an individual basis. Signs of trauma may include erythema, oedema, blisters, fissures, scabs or bruising under the skin.

A number of interventions have been recommended over the years to treat painful nipples and promote healing to maintain lactation and exclusive breastfeeding, such as ointments, sprays and nipple shields. Nipple shields have caused great controversy for many years, and many midwives are wary of suggesting them. In the past, nipple shields were promoted for mothers with sore or cracked nipples, attachment difficulties and 'flat' nipples, without trying to find out the cause of the problem first or teaching the mother about correct positioning and attachment techniques. In a multi-site, international study of 54 maternal–infant dyads using ultra-thin nipple shields, Chertok (2009) found that 89.8 per cent of mothers were satisfied in using them, and 67.3 per cent of these mothers suggested that it prevented them giving up breastfeeding. Also, there was no significant difference in weight gain for babies who fed with or without the nipple shield. This is supported by a more recent study by Coentro *et al.* (2021), who also found nipple shield use did not impact milk production or milk transfer in breastfeeding women experiencing nipple pain, suggesting the judicious use of nipple shields as a temporary measure may be helpful.

Caldwell *et al.* (2004) conducted a randomised experimental trial with 94 breastfeeding mothers with sore nipples. They randomly split these mothers into three groups: (1) those who used lanolin and breast shells, (2) those who used glycerine gel dressings and (3) those who received assessment and education on position and attachment. They found all interventions to be effective, resulting in healed nipples and decreased pain. However, all groups also included assessment and education. Therefore, the authors recommend that care for mothers with sore nipples should include assessment of position and attachment. Dennis *et al.* (2014) conducted a systematic review of good-quality studies to assess the effects of interventions in the resolution of nipple pain. They found insufficient evidence to support the use of glycerine gel dressings, breast shells with lanolin, lanolin or all-purpose ointment. In contrast, they reported that applying nothing or expressed breastmilk alone may be more beneficial in the short term.

Kent *et al.* (2015) suggested that antenatal breastfeeding education and correction of positioning and attachment in the first week after birth help prevent nipple damage and consequential cessation of breastfeeding. They also recommended early assessment to identify ankyloglossia, poor milk removal, strong infant suction and vasospasm so that appropriate treatment and management can be commenced and prevent ongoing pain and damage to the nipple.

White spot

The mother may present with a 'white spot' on the nipple and will usually complain of severe 'pin-point' breast pain. On observation of the breast a white spot can be seen on the nipple at the point of the blockage. It is thought to be an overgrowth of epithelium or build-up of fatty material (Spencer, 2008). It can be removed by gentle rubbing or piercing with a sterile needle.

Practice recommendations: nipple pain

A breastfeeding history and observation of a complete breastfeed is fundamental in determining the cause of nipple pain or trauma. The infant's sucking pattern must also be assessed to exclude tongue-tie or any other anomalies. Correct positioning and attachment must be maintained throughout the feed. The mother can be advised to position and feed the infant with the wound at the corner of the infant's mouth to avoid pressure. If the infant is incorrectly attached, the vacuum seal should be released by the mother inserting her clean finger into the corner of the infant's mouth with a little downward pressure. Pulling the infant from the breast without releasing the vacuum will cause further trauma to the nipple. If the nipple is too painful to feed, advise the mother to express breastmilk from the affected side and offer the other breast until she can resume breastfeeding from both sides.

Bacterial infection may occur if there is a break in the skin and lead to delayed wound healing and needs treatment with antibiotics. Mothers may complain of deep breast pain, and this must not be confused with thrush.

Insufficient milk supply

A common concern for breastfeeding mothers is whether their babies are getting enough milk. This is often due to a lack of confidence as a result of influences inherent in a bottle-feeding culture, where the amounts of formula milk are measured and regulated. Insufficient milk supply is often cited by mothers as a reason for early weaning or giving up breastfeeding (McAndrew *et al.*, 2012; SG, 2017; Rozga *et al.*, 2014). The role of the healthcare professional is therefore crucial in recognising the difference between perceived insufficient milk supply or physiologically delayed or failed lactogenesis to ensure mothers have the tools to give them confidence to rectify the problem and continue breastfeeding.

Physical, psychological and social factors can affect lactogenesis. Failed lactation can be classified as primary or secondary:

- **Primary** inability to produce breastmilk.
- **Secondary** due to poor techniques or management of breastfeeding problems.

Some common causes of failed lactation are hormonal imbalance due to conditions such as diabetes (Doughty and Taylor, 2021), hypothyroidism and obesity (Hurst, 2007; Preusting *et al.*, 2017). Birthing complications such as preterm birth, caesarean section and retained placenta may also be contributing factors. Other issues that may cause problems are breast trauma, surgery, anxiety or stress, postpartum haemorrhage leading to Sheehan's syndrome, and polycystic ovaries. However, failed lactogenesis is most commonly associated with a lack of skin-to-skin contact, infrequent feeding and ineffective removal of milk from the breast for a variety of reasons, such as tongue-tie, maternal–infant separation, poor attachment, supplementary feeds, and use of teats and pacifiers. The combined contraceptive pill and other medications can also inhibit milk production. This list is by no means exhaustive, and these and other issues are further discussed throughout this book.

Hurst (2007) suggested that the presence of two or more of the following risk factors for delay or failure of lactation should indicate close surveillance of the initiation of breastfeeding for signs of adequate milk supply and transfer, such as frequent wet nappies and changing stool (see Chapter 4). Signs of inadequate milk transfer are:

- Fewer than three wet nappies per day by the third day.
- Fewer than five wet nappies per day by the fourth to sixth day.
- No evidence of 'changing' stools by the third or fourth day.
- Weight loss of greater than 10 per cent of the birth weight in early days of life or not returned to birth weight by 3 weeks of age (NICE, 2018b).
- Infant not satiated.
- Soft breasts.
- No signs of milk transfer during feed (swallowing signs, visible milk).
- Persistent jaundice.

Recognising the problem at an early stage is crucial and the first steps in supporting mothers with any problems associated with breastfeeding are:

- To observe a complete breastfeed (see Chapter 4).
- To take a breastfeeding history and assessment:
    - Frequency of feeds and feeding pattern.
    - Use of supplementary feeds, teats or dummies.
    - Birth history.
    - Number of wet nappies and consistency/colour of stools.

Once the reason for the inadequate milk supply has been identified, a plan of action can be developed, implemented and evaluated. The focus of this plan should be to ensure adequate nutrition for the infant and to increase breast stimulation and effective emptying of breastmilk. This can be achieved by:

1 Skin-to-skin contact
2 Increasing the number of times the mother breastfeeds per day, ensuring at least one feed during the night. 'Switch' feeding may keep the infant awake (changing from one breast to the other several times during a feed on a short-term basis)
3 Ideally giving breastmilk, rather than formula milk, following a breastfeed if supplementation is required because of failure to thrive. This should be delivered using devices other than a bottle or teat to avoid nipple–teat confusion (see Chapter 9)
4 Teaching the mother to correct any positioning and attachment problems (see Chapter 4)
5 Rectifying any problems such as tongue-tie (see Chapter 8)
6 Additional breast stimulation and complete breast emptying using a mechanical breast pump (see Chapter 4)
7 Use of galactagogues such as domperidone and metoclopramide to increase prolactin levels, if required (see Chapter 8)

Inverted nipples

Inverted or 'flat' nipples should not affect breastfeeding because with correct positioning and attachment, the infant latches on to the breast not the nipple. However, many mothers do find inverted or flat nipples a challenge, as do midwives and health visitors when trying to support and advise them. It is important to reassure these mothers that it is possible to successfully breastfeed with inverted nipples, but they may require additional support. If it protrudes, it is not a true inverted nipple. Han and Hong (1999) classified inverted nipples as follows:

- **Grade I:** There is minimal fibrosis, and the nipple can be easily pulled out and maintain protrusion.
- **Grade II:** There is moderate fibrosis beneath the nipple. It can be pulled out but retracts.
- **Grade III:** There are severe fibrosis, and it is difficult to pull out the nipple.

Breast engorgement

Engorgement of the breasts is most often associated with delayed or infrequent feeding or with ineffective removal of the breastmilk. Engorgement is often confused with breast fullness, which occurs in the early days due to increased prolactin levels, increased blood flow to the breast and an increase in milk volume (see Table 6.1).

The engorgement can extend from the breast to include the areola and nipple, and sometimes the mother may experience a low-grade pyrexia. The mother may also complain of pain, particularly before a feed and during the night.

If engorgement is not resolved and the milk storage capacity of the breast is exceeded, it can cause the over-distension of the milk-secreting cells, altering their shape, which will decrease further milk production. If there is a build-up of breastmilk and the feedback inhibitor of lactation (FIL), this will also contribute to a decrease in milk production (see Chapter 3). The congestion can also inhibit lymphatic drainage of toxins and bacteria and predispose the mother to mastitis.

Practice recommendations: inverted nipples

There is no evidence to suggest that antenatal preparation of the nipples is effective in bringing out the nipple, but following birth, a number of practices may help mothers with inverted nipples successfully breastfeed. First, it is important to promote confidence and reassurance that the mother can breastfeed, and prolonged skin-to-skin contact will encourage breastfeeding behaviour in both mother and infant (Moore *et al.*, 2016). While establishing breastfeeding, she may need to express milk to ensure an adequate milk supply. If the breast is full and taut and the infant is having difficulty taking the breast into his or her mouth, it may be helpful to hand express a small amount of milk to soften the breast. Other techniques that may also help to protrude the nipple include:

- Encourage skin-to-skin contact.
- Teach the mother to pull out the nipple and gently roll it before feeds or to place it between the thumb and the index finger and push backwards to help it protrude.

- Use a breastmilk pump or 'nipplette' prior to breastfeeding to bring out the nipple to enable the infant to latch on to the breast more effectively.
- Assess for correct positioning and attachment. Suggest positions that aid gravity to enable the infant to scoop a mouthful of breast. If the mother is sat upright or flat, this will not help the protrusion of the nipples.
- As a last resort, some mothers may need to use nipple shields during the feed as a temporary measure.

Table 6.1 The difference between breast fullness and engorgement

Breast fullness (normal)	Engorgement (not normal)
Warm	Hot
Tender	Painful
Full	Full
Skin: possible marbling	Shiny, possibly inflamed
Milk flows	Milk does not flow easily Engorgement involves:
	• Congestion and increased vascularity
	• Accumulation of milk
	• Oedema

The pain of engorgement can be quite distressing for mothers. Zakarija-Grkovic and Stewart (2020) conducted a systematic review to identify treatments for breast engorgement. They examined trials cabbage leaves, compresses and cold gel packs. They concluded that whilst these treatments were promising, there was still insufficient evidence to support them but suggest they were unlikely to be harmful and were soothing, inexpensive and readily available.

Practice recommendations: breast engorgement

A mother with engorgement should be encouraged and supported to empty her breasts regularly. This may mean mother-led feeding rather than responsive feeding. It is crucial at this point to observe a feed to ensure attachment is correct to prevent a decrease in milk production. If the infant is having difficulty attaching to the breast due to the fullness, it can be helpful to express a small amount of breastmilk to make the areola softer, which will make it easier for the infant to attach to the breast.

Despite a lack of evidence chilled savoy cabbage leaves are commonly recommended to sooth breast pain. The leaf is placed inside the bra over the breast for 10–15 minutes.

A warm compress prior to a feed and cold compresses following the feed may be helpful; however, some mothers will require oral analgesia such as paracetamol or ibuprofen.

Blocked ducts

Blocked ducts are usually caused by ineffective removal of breastmilk, resulting in milk stasis in the lactiferous ducts, or by restrictive clothing, such as a tight bra, causing pressure on the outside of the breast. Blocked ducts present as localised tenderness and redness in an area of the breast.

Mastitis

Mastitis is inflammation of the mammary gland. If engorgement or blocked ducts are not corrected and milk stasis persists, it may lead to mastitis and ultimately cessation of breastfeeding. Other causes of mastitis are infrequent or poor emptying of the breast; sore or cracked nipples, which can be a portal for infection; blocked milk ducts; thrush, *Candida albicans* infection; and restrictive clothing, such as a tight bra or injury (bumps and knocks). Frequent breastfeeding can reduce the risk of mothers developing mastitis (NICE, 2021b). In a Cochrane systematic review to assess preventative strategies on the occurrence and re-occurrence of mastitis, Crepinsek *et al.* (2020) found some evidence that acupoint massage is probably better than routine care and that probiotics 'show promise', but the evidence is currently incomplete. They also suggested breast massage and low-frequency pulse treatment may reduce the risk of mastitis. The evidence reviewed regarding other interventions such as breastfeeding education, pharmacological treatments and alternative therapies suggest they may be little better than routine care for preventing mastitis, but due to the low certainty of the evidence, conclusions are uncertain. However, Douglas (2022) suggested that avoidance of high intra-alveolar and intra-ductal pressure is key to prevent discontinuation of lactation. She recommended conservative management and avoidance of lump massage or vibration and other external pressures on the breast that may increase micro-vascular trauma and inflammation.

It is important to observe a complete feed to ensure attachment is correct; otherwise the duct will not be emptied, leading to further discomfort and stasis of the milk, which could develop into mastitis. If breastmilk is not effectively removed, there will be a build-up of FIL and milk production will be reduced.

Practice recommendations: blocked ducts

The following measures may be helpful:

- Breastfeed regularly and start with the affected side first to promote drainage. Avoid breasts becoming too full.
- Avoid anything that applies pressure on the nipple or breast during milk removal that will compress the lactiferous ducts (Douglas, 2022).
- Avoid lump massage or any external pressure to the breast such as constrictive clothing and breast shells, which may cause compression if the lactiferous ducts.
- Warm compresses prior to a feed and cold compresses following the feed may be helpful.
- Massage over the affected area of breast, particularly during a feed, to disperse the blockage.

- During a feed, position the infant's chin adjacent to the blocked duct to empty this area of the breast more effectively.
- Wean or discontinue breastfeeding gradually.

Mastitis is usually unilateral, affecting one or two ducts, but can also be seen in both breasts. Mastitis is an inflammatory response to breastmilk's leaking into the tissue from a blocked duct, and it may or may not involve infection (BFN, 2022). If milk stasis persists and infection ensues, it is most commonly due to *Staphylococcus aureus* (NICE, 2021b).

Mastitis is usually diagnosed clinically and presents with the following symptoms:

- erythema or inflammation of an area of the breast; a hot, red, swollen wedge-shaped area;
- breast pain; and
- 'flu-like' symptoms, including fever (temperature in excess of 38.4°C), headache, fatigue and general aches and pains in response to the inflammatory process.

It is not possible to diagnose infectious or non-infectious mastitis but it may be more likely to be infectious if there is a fissure on the nipple or if symptoms do not improve within 12–24 hours or worsen or positive bacterial culture in breastmilk (NICE, 2021b).

Collecting a specimen of breastmilk

If a specimen of breastmilk for culture is required, the correct technique for taking it should be explained to the mothers. She should wash her hands and clean her breast before expressing a small amount of breastmilk. This should then be discarded. She should then express some more breastmilk into a sterile container, avoiding contact with the nipple and container.

Practice recommendations: mastitis

- The mother should be encouraged to continue breastfeeding more frequently than usual to ensure the breast is effectively emptied, as not doing so may exacerbate the condition. There is no risk to the infant as the mother and infant are colonised with the same organisms. However, some babies appear to dislike the taste of the milk from the affected breast, possibly due to the increased sodium content; therefore, the milk from this breast may be expressed and discarded. It is crucial to observe a feed to ensure positioning and attachment are correct and that the infant is feeding well.
- Changing positions for feeding may be helpful. Position the infant so that the chin and nose point to the affected part of the breast to assist with drainage.
- Teaching the mother to recognise the signs of an effective feed is essential so that she does not discontinue the feed prematurely or attempt to empty the breast as this may increase supply and make inflammation worse (BFN, 2022) (see Chapter 4).

- If the mother feels unable to breastfeed, she should be encouraged to express regularly. At first, the milk production may be increased; however, the mother should be reassured that this will be temporary, and the number of times she expresses can be reduced as the symptoms of mastitis subside.
- Recommend rest and increasing fluid intake.
- A warm compress or shower prior to a feed and a cold compress following the feed may be helpful.
- Give non-steroidal anti-inflammatory medications such as ibuprofen 400 mg three times a day (avoid if the mother is asthmatic or has stomach ulcers) and/ or paracetamol 1 g four times a day to reduce the pyrexia. **Aspirin should not be taken while breastfeeding** (BFN, 2022).
- A breastmilk sample for culture should be obtained if mastitis is severe or recurrent, hospital-acquired infection is possible or there is severe deep burning breast pain (NICE, 2021b).
- Antibiotics are required if symptoms persist and the mastitis is thought to be due to infection, usually flucloxacillin 500 mg with erythromycin 500 mg four times or cefalexin 250–500 mg four times a day if she is allergic to penicillin (BFN, 2022). Mothers must be informed that antibiotics may cause the infant to have a loose stool, and they must also be vigilant for thrush.

Spencer (2008) points out that mastitis resembles inflammatory breast cancer and, when mastitis does not respond to treatment as expected, this should be considered alongside other differential diagnosis (see NICE, 2021b for further detail). Admission to hospital may be required if there are:

- signs of sepsis (tachycardia, fever, chills);
- infection progresses rapidly; or
- the mother is haemodynamically unstable or immunocompromised.

In such cases, the infant should be admitted with the mother to continue breastfeeding. Referral to a general surgeon should be made if a breast abscess is suspected.

Abscesses

An abscess can be a result of mastitis caused by *Staphylococcus aureus* and needs urgent referral to a general surgeon for confirmation by ultrasound, drainage of the abscess under ultrasound and a culture taken to determine the choice of antibiotics (NICE, 2021b). Breastfeeding can continue if the mother is well enough, otherwise breastmilk must be expressed to avoid a build-up of FIL.

Ways of preventing the development of a breast abscess include:

- Effective milk removal and avoidance of milk stasis.
- Treatment of breast inflammation and infection.
- Maternal education regarding position and attachment, demand feeding and avoidance of abrupt weaning.

Thrush or *Candida albicans*

Thrush is rare in the first few weeks, and Jones (BFN, 2020) expressed concern of over-diagnosis. Diagnosing thrush can be very difficult, so before commencing treatment, it should be confirmed by swabbing the nipple and infant's mouth for fungal or bacterial infection (usually *S. aureus*). Other causes for the breast pain must also be excluded, such as poor positioning and attachment of the infant to the breast, eczema, tongue-tie, white spot, Raynaud's syndrome and infection.

Signs and symptoms in the mother

- Thrush is usually very painful. The mother often complains of a shooting pain through the breast, which begins during the breastfeed and continues for up to an hour after feeding.
- Initially, breast pain may be localised to one breast but quickly transfers to both.
- The nipple may be itchy or sensitive, or there may be a permanent loss of colour to the nipple and areola. Care must be taken not to confuse this with the temporary loss of colour caused by poor positioning and attachment or Raynaud's syndrome (poor circulation).
- There may be a delay in the healing of cracked nipples.
- The mother will have an absence of red area on the breast and pyrexia.

Signs and symptoms in the infant

- The infant may also exhibit signs of oral thrush (white plaques on the tongue that do not rub away) or nappy rash.
- The infant may keep pulling off the breast, possibly due to a sore mouth or poor attachment, and may be windy and unsettled after a breastfeed.

Practice recommendations: thrush

A full breastfeeding history, assessment and observation of a feed are essential to rule out problems other than thrush before prescribing medication. The Breastfeeding Network (2020) discourages the use of medication until positioning and attachment have been observed by a skilled practitioner. Mothers should be encouraged to continue feeding to avoid a build-up of the FIL and milk stasis. If they have any frozen breastmilk, it may be best to discard it to prevent reinfection.

Following diagnosis of thrush, simultaneous treatment is required, including nipple and oral treatment for the mother where there is severe or deep breast pain and the infant's mouth:

- **Mother:** Miconazole 2% gel should be used on the nipple and areola; apply sparingly. Gel is not recommended. When oral treatment is required, fluconazole 150–400 mg loading dose followed by 100–200 mg twice a day for ten days is recommended but not licensed for use in lactating women (BFN, 2020). If nipples are red or inflamed, hydrocortisone 1% may be considered in addition (NICE, 2022a).

- **Infant:** Miconazole gel should be applied inside the mouth, with a clean finger, four times a day: 1 ml for 0–1 month and 2.5 mls for over 1 month. Do not apply with a spoon due to the risk of choking. Caution must be taken as the manufacturer does not license this product for infants under 4 months old, and with care for 4–6 months old. The problem is thought to be with the application of the gel rather than the medication (BFN, 2020).

Up-to-date information for medical treatment is also available from Thrush (of the breast/nipple) and Breastfeeding – The Breastfeeding Network.

Symptoms should subside in two or three days, but if they have not resolved within seven days, the general practitioner should be informed.

Mothers should also be advised of other measures that can be helpful (BFN, 2020), such as:

- Following a feed, the breast should be gently rinsed with clear water to remove milk residue.
- Hands should be washed before a breastfeed and following nappy changes.
- Analgesia, such as paracetamol and ibuprofen, should be administered.
- Each member of the family should use a separate towel as it can be passed between family members.
- Any dummies, teats and nipple shields should be sterilised, preferably by boiling for 20 minutes, as they are a common cause of reinfection.
- Probiotics may be helpful as well as reducing the level of yeast and sugar in the diet as well as acidophilus capsules to restore healthy bacteria.

Concluding comments

Many of the common problems of breastfeeding stem from poor positioning and attachment, and it is therefore crucial that mothers are taught how to do this correctly and how to recognise an effective breastfeed. UNICEF UK BFI recommends that a minimum of two breastfeeding assessments be carried out in the first week followed by a plan of care. They have developed checklists to help midwives, neonatal nurses and health visitors as well as mothers recognise that the baby is feeding well. These can be found at www.unicef.org.uk/BabyFriendly/Resources.

The key areas to remember when addressing breastfeeding problems are:

- Carry out a breastfeeding assessment.
- Observe a complete breastfeed for effective milk transfer, correct position and attachment and sucking pattern.
- Observe for breast or nipple anomalies.
- Assess the infant's mouth for tongue-tie or any other anomaly.
- Encourage skin-to-skin contact.
- Use positive language to promote confidence.
- Produce a care plan to avoid conflicting advice.

Chapters, 7 and 8 explore more specific issues when the mother or infant have special needs that require more specialist advice.

Scenarios

How would you manage the following situations, and what advice would you give?

1 On the tenth postnatal day, Daisy tells you she has a cracked right nipple, and it is very painful when feeding. She has stopped feeding from that side to let it heal.
2 Alison gave birth to Eve ten days ago following a traumatic forceps delivery and postpartum haemorrhage of 1,000 ml. When you visit, Alison tells you that Eve is not settling, and she does not think she has enough breastmilk and is thinking about changing to formula.
3 Bridget's partner phones you to ask you to visit because Bridget is unwell and has a very painful, red left breast that is hot to the touch. When you arrive, she has flu-like symptoms and is in a lot of pain. She has been reluctant to take any medication because she is breastfeeding.

Resources

- Breastfeeding Network (BFN)
  www.breastfeedingnetwork.org.uk/

- Cochrane Library
  www.thecochranelibrary.com

- La Leche League
  www.laleche.org.uk

- NICE Clinical Knowledge Summaries
  cks.nice.org.uk/breastfeeding-problems

7 Supporting mothers with special needs

- Learning outcomes
- Human immunodeficiency virus
- Herpes simplex virus type 1
- Hepatitis B
- Hepatitis C
- Tuberculosis
- COVID-19
- Substance misuse
- Delayed lactogenesis
- Caesarean section
- Diabetes
- Obesity
- Polycystic ovary syndrome
- Postpartum haemorrhage
- Breast surgery and anomalies
- Epilepsy
- Hyperlactation or galactorrhea
- Twins
- Concluding comments
- Scenario
- Further reading
- Resources

Most mothers have the ability to breastfeed successfully for the first six months following birth and to continue beyond this, alongside solid food, up to two years and beyond, as recommended by the WHO (2021a). However, a small number of mothers may be unable to breastfeed or may have difficulty initiating and maintaining lactation and require a great deal of support and advice from midwives and health visitors; some may temporarily need to supplement breastfeeding or use breastmilk substitutes. The

DOI: 10.4324/9781003282341-7

WHO and UNICEF UK Baby Friendly Initiative (BFI) (2009, pp. 8–9) published a list of acceptable medical reasons for temporary or long-term use of breastmilk substitutes:

- **Maternal conditions that may justify permanent avoidance of breastfeeding:**

  - Human immunodeficiency virus (HIV) infection if replacement feeding is acceptable, feasible, affordable, sustainable and safe.

- **Maternal conditions that may justify temporary avoidance of breastfeeding:**

  - Severe illness that prevents a mother from caring for her infant, for example, sepsis.
  - Herpes simplex virus type 1 (HSV-1).
  - Maternal medication:

    - Sedating psychotherapeutic drugs, anti-epileptic drugs and opioids may cause side effects such as drowsiness and respiratory depression and are better avoided if a safer alternative is available.
    - Radioactive iodine-131 is best avoided. Breastfeeding can resume two months after receiving this substance.
    - Excessive topical iodine or iodophors can result in thyroid suppression and electrolyte abnormalities.
    - Cytotoxic chemotherapy.

- **Maternal conditions during which breastfeeding can still continue, although health problems may be of concern:**

  - Breast abscess: Breastfeeding can continue on the unaffected side and resume on the affected side once treatment has commenced; however, milk must be expressed to prevent exacerbation of the condition (see Chapter 6).
  - Mastitis can be very painful; however, milk must be expressed to prevent exacerbation of the condition (see Chapter 6).
  - Hepatitis B: Infants should be given the hepatitis B vaccine within 48 hours of birth or as soon as possible thereafter.
  - Tuberculosis (TB).
  - Substance use: Mothers should be encouraged to avoid the following and given support and advice to abstain:

    - Nicotine, alcohol, ecstasy, amphetamines, cocaine and other stimulants have demonstrated harmful effects.
    - Alcohol, opioids, benzodiazepines and cannabis can cause sedation in both the mother and infant.

This chapter focuses on the issues related to mothers with special needs and some other conditions or situations that may also pose problems and challenges with breastfeeding. Chapter 8 discusses issues related to infants with special needs.

Learning outcomes

By the end of this chapter, you will be able to:

- describe the advice that should be given to HIV-positive mothers in the UK;

- identify those conditions or situations where breastfeeding may be temporarily challenged; and
- provide evidence-based information for mothers to help them maintain lactation.

Mapping to UNICEF Baby Friendly Initiative (BFI) Education learning outcomes (2019a)

By the end of the programme, students will:

Theme		Learning outcomes
Theme 2: Support infant feeding	6.	Have the knowledge and skills to support mothers and babies to maximise breastmilk and breastfeeding, to continue to breastfeed for as long as they wish and to introduce solid foods at an appropriate time.
Theme 4: Managing the challenges	11.	Be able to apply their knowledge of the physiology of lactation and infant feeding to support effective management of challenges which may arise at any time during breastfeeding.
	12.	Have an understanding of the special circumstances which can affect lactation and breastfeeding (e.g. when mother and baby are separated, including preterm and sick infants) and be able to support mothers to overcome the challenges.
Theme 5: Promote positive communication	14.	Have an understanding of the principles of effective communication and current thinking around public health promotion strategies and approaches.

Human immunodeficiency virus

Human immunodeficiency virus (HIV) and breastfeeding continue to be debated, but in the UK, it is recommended on the www.nhs.uk website that bottle feeding rather than breastfeeding is a way to reduce passing HIV to the infant. However, they go on to say that the chances of passing HIV through breastmilk are lower if the HIV viral load is undetectable and the mother is taking antiretroviral (ARV) drugs. In this situation, if the mother chooses to breastfeed, regular checks are offered to monitor any transmission. The advice is clear: 'do not breastfeed your baby if your viral load is detectable'. Much of the evidence around breastfeeding with HIV comes from studies carried out in developing countries and may not be applicable to mothers in the UK and other countries where the problems associated with formula feeding do not exist (Raina and Preston, 2014).

It is the role of healthcare professionals to provide HIV-positive mothers with information so they can make informed choices regarding infant feeding. Therefore, all mothers should be offered an HIV test as part of the antenatal care programme, as well as information about HIV during pregnancy and the implications for the infant.

The most common way children are infected by HIV is through vertical transmission before, during or after birth when breastfeeding. This risk is reduced to 1 in 100 with treatment by a combination therapy of highly active antiretroviral (HAART) drugs, even if the mother does not require it for her own health status. Birth by caesarean section is recommended if the mother is not taking combination therapy or if there is a detectable viral load (www.nhs.uk). If the mother becomes infected with HIV during breastfeeding, the risk of vertical transmission is greater due to the high viral load than if she was previously infected. Therefore, mothers at risk of acquiring HIV should receive advice on reducing the risk.

Spencer (2008) suggested transmission of HIV is more likely if the mother has mastitis or cracked nipples. Breastfeeding mothers should be taught how to avoid developing mastitis and cracked nipples, but if they do occur, they should not breastfeed from the affected breast and instead regularly express breastmilk, ensuring the breast is effectively emptied to prevent cessation of milk production.

In 2010, the World Health Organization (WHO) developed guidelines stating HIV-infected mothers should not breastfeed where replacement feeding is acceptable in the society and if parents can afford formula and sustain it for six months, which includes having access to appropriate facilities to prepare formula safely, in hygienic conditions, with safe water. Where this is not possible, the WHO recommends that breastfeeding should continue exclusively for six months and alongside the introduction of other foods up to 12 months of age, provided the mother and/or infant continue to take the antiretroviral drugs, which they suggest the mother should commence at 14 weeks' gestation. Evidence demonstrates that with strict adherence to the antiretroviral regimen in pregnancy and during breastfeeding, the HIV infection rate may be as low as 2 per cent (WHO, 2010). Unfortunately, some mothers and infants do not have access to these medications and are advised to breastfeed exclusively for no more than the first six months of life and then abruptly wean, introducing a breastmilk substitute along with solid foods. This guidance was updated in 2013 and again in 2016. Whilst the 2016 update acknowledged that the 2010 guidance remained valid, the following revisions were made:

- Mothers living with HIV should breastfeed for at least 12 months and may continue for up to 24 months or longer while fully supported on antiretroviral therapy (ART) (WHO, 2016, p. 3).
- Mothers living with HIV can be reassured that ART reduces the risk of postnatal transmission in the context of mixed feeding. Although exclusive breastfeeding is recommended, practicing mixed feeding is not a reason to stop breastfeeding in the presence of ARV drugs (WHO, 2016, p. 4).

The issue of infant feeding should be raised as early as possible with HIV-positive mothers and those at risk, and it will be the mother's informed decision how she intends to feed. Either way, parents will need support and advice: for breastfeeding mothers, how to avoid the risks of vertical transmission and for those who choose to formula-feed how to safely make up a feed and sterilise equipment.

The rest of this chapter focuses on situations in which breastfeeding is challenging.

Herpes simplex virus type 1

HSV-1 is the virus that normally causes cold sores around the mouth and genital herpes but in newborns can affect the immune system. Although HSV-1 can be found in the breastmilk of symptomatic mothers, there is no evidence to suggest vertical transmission is a problem. However, HSV-1 can be transmitted by direct contact, and therefore direct contact between the lesions on the mother's breasts or mouth and the infant should be avoided (D'Andrea and Spatz, 2019). This may have implications for skin-to-skin contact. If the lesions are on the breast, feeding from that side should be avoided until it has cleared up. Nevertheless, the breast must be regularly emptied by expression to avoid a build-up of feedback inhibitor of lactation (FIL) and to maintain the milk supply in the affected breast; the expressed milk should be discarded. Feeding from the unaffected side can continue as normal. Antiviral drugs such as acyclovir can be prescribed and are safe during breastfeeding (BFN, 2019b). Mothers should also be educated about the importance of hand washing, washing of blankets and towels, and avoiding kissing the infant if the lesions are on the mouth.

Hepatitis B

Hepatitis B is a serious liver infection that can cause liver failure or cirrhosis. It is transmitted via infected blood and other body fluids. Specialist Pharmacy Service (SPS, 2020) advises that women with hepatitis B can breastfeed and there is no risk of transmission. Infants of mothers who test positive for hepatitis B should be given hepatitis B vaccine and hepatitis B immune globulin as soon as possible, preferably within the first 24 hours of life (Hepatitis B Foundation, 2020). The Hepatitis B Foundation (2020) recommends breastfeeding for infants who are immunised as the benefits outweigh the potential risk of infection.

Hepatitis C

Hepatitis C is a disease of the liver caused by the hepatitis C virus (HCV), which may develop into cirrhosis of the liver, liver failure or liver cancer. There is no vaccine for HCV. It is a blood-borne virus, but SPS (2020) advises breastfeeding is not contraindicated as long as the mother is HIV negative.

Tuberculosis

Mothers at risk for TB are those who have been in an area where it is endemic or in close contact with someone who has the active disease. Women who are HIV positive or are immunosuppressed are also at risk. The risk to the fetus in utero is minimal, and if treated, the prognosis is good. However, if untreated, the newborn can become infected through close contact with the mother. Screening for TB should be offered to those at risk (e.g. through recent exposure to TB or being HIV positive).

TB is not transmitted through breastmilk. Mothers infected with TB and taking treatment can breastfeed because the concentrations of the medication in breastmilk are too small to be toxic. Mothers taking isoniazid should also take 10–25 mg pyridoxine (vitamin B6) supplementation daily (PHE, 2019).

COVID-19

COVID-19 first presented in China in late 2019 and by January 2020 was identified as a novel coronavirus, severe acute respiratory syndrome coronavirus 2 (SARS-CoV-2). In March 2020, the WHO declared a pandemic. Due to the lack of evidence initially, there was a lot of confusion on the guidance to be given to breastfeeding mothers, and many advised to discontinue breastfeeding as it is primarily transmitted by person-to-person spread through respiratory aerosols. However, as evidence emerged, it was clear that COVID-19 is not a contraindication to breastfeeding, and therefore breastfeeding should be recommended as usual (WHO, 2020; RCOG/RCM, 2022; BAPM, 2022). WHO (2020, p. 1) suggests the development of any recommendations consider 'the potential risks of COVID-19 infection of the infant, but also the risks of morbidity and mortality associated with not breastfeeding, the inappropriate use of infant formula milks, as well as the protective effects of skin-to-skin contact'.

Perinatal transmission of COVID-19 is rare and appears to result in minor illness in young infants, or they may be asymptomatic (BAPM, 2022). WHO (2020) recommend mothers and babies should continue to have skin-to skin contact and stay together whether they have suspected or confirmed COVID-19. Krogstad *et al.* (2022) found no evidence to suggest breastfeeding poses a risk of transmission of SARS-CoV-2 RNA for infants. They examined breastmilk from 110 lactating women following recent infection and found no evidence of SARS-CoV-2 RNA in breastmilk. However, many mothers have concerns and should be offered the opportunity talk to a professional who will listen and provide evidence-based information that the benefits of breastfeeding outweigh the risk of transmission. UNICEF UK BFI has produced a series of guidance for healthcare professionals to help guide these conversations, including where remote support is required. Some common challenges are included (see www.unicef.org.uk/babyfriendly).

To limit spread of the virus to infants, the British Association of Perinatal Medicine recommends:

- Wash hands before touching the baby, breast pump or bottles.
- Avoid coughing or sneezing on the baby while feeding.
- Consider wearing a face covering or fluid-resistant facemask while feeding or caring for the baby. Babies should not wear masks or other face coverings as they may risk suffocation.

UNICEF BFI suggest that when asymptomatic, it is important to encourage interaction with infants without wearing a mask. If the mother is unwell and unable to breastfeed, she should be supported to maintain lactation and express breastmilk or be offered donor breastmilk to give by an alternative method (see Chapter 9). In addition, if in hospital, a dedicated breast pump should be provided. For mothers who chose to bottle feed, it is important to adhere to sterilisation guidance (see Chapter 9).

Emerging evidence suggest the risk of separating mother and infant and not breastfeeding is greater than the risk of transmitting the virus. There is also suggestion that breastmilk from a mother testing positive for COVID-19 may protect the infant from infection.

Vaccinations

Advice from the Joint Committee on Vaccination and Immunisation (JCVI) is that pregnant women are more at risk of severe COVID-19 disease and have been offered the vaccination and subsequent boosters in line with recommendations from the WHO. The JCVI also recommend that the vaccines can be received whilst breastfeeding. The Royal College of Obstetricians and Gynaecologists (RCOG, November 2022) stated that whilst emerging research suggests there may be trace amounts of the vaccine detected briefly in breastmilk following vaccination, reports are inconsistent, and no vaccine mRNA has been identified in infants of mothers who have been vaccinated. In addition, they state COVID-19 vaccination remains the best way to protect both mothers and their infants from COVID-19, and there are good data showing no adverse effects on babies following maternal vaccination. Breastfeeding should continue as normal following vaccination.

The COVID-19 pandemic highlighted the concerns parents have about breastfeeding and having other vaccinations. The Breastfeeding Network advises that neither activated nor live vaccines affect the safety of breastfeeding, and breastfeeding is not a contraindication for any UK-licensed vaccines. They provide a comprehensive summary of the common vaccinations in the UK (www.breastfeedingnetwork.org.uk/vaccinations).

Substance misuse

Substance misuse and breastfeeding is a contentious issue, and healthcare professionals need to weigh up the risk–benefit ratio when advising mothers about the benefits of breastfeeding; however, this may be difficult because there is limited research in this area. The DHSC (2017) guidance encourages breastfeeding with exceptions to this advice for mothers taking large amounts stimulants such as cocaine, amphetamines, methamphetamine or benzodiazepines, when breastfeeding is contraindicated (WHO, 2014b; DHSC, 2017; Wilson *et al.*, 2020). WHO (2014b, p. 15) recommends:

- Mothers with substance use disorders should be encouraged to breastfeed unless the risks outweigh the benefits.
- Breastfeeding women using alcohol or drugs should be advised and supported to cease alcohol or drug use; however, substance use is not necessarily a contraindication to breastfeeding.
  - Skin-to skin contact is important regardless of feeding choice and needs to be actively encouraged for a mother with a substance use disorder who is able to respond to her baby's needs.
  - Mothers who are stable on opioid maintenance treatment with either methadone or buprenorphine should be encouraged to breastfeed unless the risks clearly outweigh the benefits.

Most drugs are transferred to the infant through breastmilk. WHO (2014b) suggests breastfeeding may reduce the severity of withdrawal symptoms in infants. McCrory and Richens (2007, p. 206) describe it as a 'theoretical situation'; because the infant is getting some of the drug, it could be considered unadvisable, but in reality, the fetus is getting larger amounts in utero. These infants are vulnerable and are at higher risk of sudden infant death syndrome (SIDS), poor nutrition and weight gain due to the chaotic lifestyle their mothers often lead; therefore, the benefits of breastfeeding may outweigh the negative effects of the drug abuse and lifestyle. Cannabis use is thought to suppress the production of prolactin and causes many of the problems associated with smoking because it is usually combined with tobacco; it is therefore advisable to avoid breastfeeding for several hours after smoking it. Effects on infants are unclear, but it is thought to cause drowsiness, poor feeding and developmental delay and due to the uncertainty about long term outcomes should be discouraged (National Institute on Drug Abuse (NIDA), 2020).

Dryden *et al.* (2009) conducted a retrospective cohort study of 450 drug-dependent women from an inner-city hospital to investigate factors associated with the development of neonatal abstinence syndrome (NAS) and the implications for healthcare resources. They found that infants who were breastfed for more than 72 hours were less likely to require treatment for NAS. They suggested this could be due to the benefits of breastmilk combined with the small traces of drug in the breastmilk lessening withdrawal symptoms, and the soothing effect of breastfeeding. They recommend these mothers should have an increased length of postnatal stay in hospital and increased support to continue breastfeeding while observing for signs of NAS in the infant. Jambert-Gray *et al.* (2009) support these findings and highlight the importance of breastfeeding to improving self-esteem and suggest that these mothers may be more likely to wean themselves off methadone.

Smoking

Although smoking while breastfeeding is not recommended, the benefits of breastmilk outweigh the risks from nicotine. Dorea stated that it is 'worse to smoke and not breastfeed' (2007, p. 290). Nicotine is found in breastmilk and alters the taste (NIDA, 2020). Mothers who smoke have a reduced milk supply and have a shorter duration of breastfeeding than their counterparts (Napierala *et al.*, 2016). It is proposed that nicotine inhibits the production of prolactin; however, further research is required in this area. Excessive crying, fussiness and colic in infants of mothers who smoke are reported, which may lead to cessation of breastfeeding because of the mothers' perception of insufficient milk supply (Giglia *et al.*, 2006; BFN, 2019c).

During pregnancy, all mothers who smoke should be offered support and help to stop smoking and, where available, referral to a smoking cessation practitioner who will provide advice on how to give up or reduce smoking. Nicotine replacement therapy is thought to decrease the amount of nicotine transferred in breastmilk. If the mother chooses to continue to smoke while breastfeeding, she should be advised not to smoke before a feed but afterwards because it takes approximately 95 minutes for nicotine to be cleared from breastmilk, with levels peaking 30–60 minutes after smoking a cigarette (BFN, 2019c). She should also be encouraged to smoke away from the infant as passive smoking is also a risk factor for SIDS, respiratory infections and asthma.

Alcohol

In recent years, recommendations about alcohol consumption while breastfeeding have been confusing for mothers and professionals alike because of a lack of robust research. Alcohol does pass into breastmilk and affects the smell and taste. Current NHS UK guidelines (2022) suggest that an occasional drink is unlikely to harm an infant, especially if the mother waits at least two hours after having a drink to feed the infant (BFN, 2021). In the past, mothers were erroneously advised to drink alcohol to increase their milk production. This may have been because alcohol can increase prolactin levels immediately, but after an hour of consumption, the levels are decreased, as is milk yield (Menella and Pepino, 2008). It also has a negative effect on oxytocin and milk ejection. Because of the lack of conclusive research, many mothers may choose not to drink alcohol at all while breastfeeding.

Practice recommendations: substance misuse

- Avoid separation; if treatment for NAS is required, it can be done on the postnatal ward.
- Prolong skin-to-skin contact to encourage breastfeeding and bonding, to regulate the infant's heart and respiratory rate and temperature and to reduce crying and sooth irritability.
- If there is separation, encourage regular expression of breastmilk.

To minimise harm:

- Discourage injection of drugs because of the risk of transmitting HIV.
- Breastfeed immediately before drug use.
- Express before drug use so that breastmilk is available.
- Monitor the infant for signs of NAS.
- Do not sleep with the infant in bed or on the settee.

However, if a mother chooses to drink alcohol, it should be avoided before a feed, as it takes approximately two hours to clear alcohol (one standard drink) from the breastmilk, and peak levels appear at approximately 30–90 minutes following intake (BFN, 2021) and four to eight hours after consuming more than one standard drink in a single occasion (WHO, 2014b). As feeding is unpredictable, some mothers choose to plan when they are going to consume alcohol and express milk to feed their infants.

Key fact

Breastfeeding mothers can eat peanuts while breastfeeding as part of a healthy balanced diet unless they are allergic to them (see www.nhs.uk).

Delayed lactogenesis

Lactogenesis II is the onset of milk production and occurs following expulsion of the placenta and membranes, which results in a sudden drop in progesterone and oestrogen levels (neuroendocrine control). As prolactin levels increase, it binds with prolactin receptors in the walls of the lactocytes and begins milk synthesis. Skin-to-skin contact at birth with the infant stimulates the production of prolactin and oxytocin. Early and regular breastfeeding inhibits the production of the prolactin-inhibiting factor (PIF) and stimulates production of prolactin. Lactogenesis II commences 30–40 hours after birth, but mothers do not feel the milk 'coming in' until about 2–3 days after birth (see Chapter 3).

Lactogenesis III is the autocrine regulation where supply and demand regulate milk production. A whey protein called FIL is secreted by the lactocytes. As the alveoli distend, there is a build-up of FIL, and milk synthesis is inhibited. When the breastmilk is effectively removed and the concentrations of FIL reduce, milk synthesis resumes. This is a local mechanism and can occur in one or both breasts. It exerts a negative feedback response to inhibit milk production when there is ineffective removal of breastmilk from the breast (see Chapter 3).

Mothers who experience delayed onset of lactogenesis II are more likely to have a shorter duration of breastfeeding and therefore need a lot of support and encouragement. The most common reason for delayed lactogenesis II is ineffective removal of milk from the breast, usually due to poor position and attachment or delayed suckling. However, there may be certain factors that inhibit effective removal of breastmilk or influence delay of lactogenesis II such as:

Breast surgery	Retained products of conception	Anxiety and lack of confidence
Obesity	Polycystic ovaries	Caesarean section
Hormonal problems	Diabetes	Preterm birth

(Dewey *et al.*, 2005)

Some of these factors are discussed further in this chapter and in Chapter 8, but the plan of care for any condition or problem that may result in delayed lactogenesis should follow the same main principles to encourage lactation:

- skin-to-skin contact;
- early and regular feeding or expression;
- avoiding separation of mother and infant when possible; and
- regular assessment of milk transfer.

Caesarean section

Following caesarean section, mothers are at risk of delayed lactation and a shortened duration of breastfeeding (Li *et al.*, 2021). Baxter (2006) conducted a quantitative survey of 422 women in England who had given birth by caesarean section, with a 65 per cent response rate, to explore their experiences of breastfeeding. She found that 84 per cent of the sample commenced breastfeeding, of whom 65 per cent were still breast-feeding between five and eight weeks after giving birth. The most common reason for giving up breastfeeding was the perception of insufficient milk and inconvenience. Other reasons cited were lack of support, difficulty with attachment and pain.

Key fact

Caffeine is transferred in breastmilk and may keep breastfeeding infants awake and cause irritability. It is therefore advisable to avoid food and drinks containing caffeine (tea, coffee, chocolate) and when possible or to limit caffeine intake to 200 mg per day (100 mg caffeine in a mug of instant coffee). Caffeine levels peak one hour after consumption. Iron levels in breastmilk are reduced when drinking more than three cups of coffee a day.

Hospital practices following a caesarean section may inhibit lactation. Stevens *et al.* (2014) conducted a review of the literature and found that skin-to-skin contact immediately after caesarean section increased breastfeeding initiation, bonding and maternal satisfaction and reduced formula supplementation, as well as provided other benefits of skin contact such as stabilising temperature. Gregson *et al.* (2016) identified a correlation between length of time of skin-to-skin contact and duration of breastfeeding. Following a caesarean section, mothers will have intravenous infusions, a catheter and pain from the scar site. Therefore, it is particularly important to assist the mother following caesarean section in practical issues such as easy access to the infant and ensuring she is in a comfortable position to attach her infant to the breast.

Most caesarean section incisions are now in the lower segment of the uterus, thus making it difficult to hold the infant in the cradle position. Other suggested positions for breastfeeding are the mother lying on her side, the 'underarm' hold or putting a pillow over her lap to place the baby on to avoid pressure on her scar.

The Association of Anaesthetists of Great Britain and Ireland (Mitchell *et al.*, 2020) published a review of the pharmacokinetics of drugs used during anaesthesia in response to regular interruption of breastfeeding and inconsistent advice from professionals. They advise mothers should be supported to breastfeed after surgery and anaesthesia once they are alert and able to feed without the need to discard breastmilk.

Practice recommendations: caesarean section

- Skin-to-skin contact in theatre if possible and to continue as long as possible. If the mother is unable to provide skin-to-skin contact, the father should be encouraged to do so.
- Early and regular breastfeeding or regular expressing should be done eight to ten times a day to promote lactation. To ensure lactation is adequate, there should be careful assessment of the infant's hydration, wet nappies and changing stool, and signs of jaundice.
- If separated, ensure a visit is arranged as soon as possible and encourage expressing in front of the infant to aid the let-down reflex.
- Ensure the environment is conducive to breastfeeding and provide ongoing skilled support, particularly with positioning and attachment.

Diabetes

There are three types of diabetes breastfeeding mothers may have:

- Type 1 diabetes (insulin-dependent diabetes – beta cells of the pancreas do not produce insulin).
- Type 2 diabetes (non-insulin diabetes – metabolic disorder, associated with obesity; insulin is present, but receptor cells do not respond).
- Gestational diabetes (glucose intolerance developed in pregnancy).

Infants born to mothers with diabetes are at greater risk of prematurity, macrosomia, birth by caesarean section, respiratory problems, congenital abnormalities, hypocalcaemia, polycythaemia and hyperbilirubinaemia (Doughty and Taylor, 2021). Following birth, newborns are also at greater risk of hypoglycaemia because of maternal hyperinsulinism in pregnancy, resulting in neonatal hypoglycaemia. Chertok *et al.* (2009) demonstrated higher blood glucose levels in infants who were breastfed within the first 30 minutes of birth compared with those who did not receive an early breast or received artificial milk for the first feed.

Bortoli and Amir (2021) conducted a systematic review to determine if mothers with diabetes in pregnancy have a delayed onset of lactation. They concluded that there was evidence of an association, but there are also many other confounding factors known to be risk factors associated to diabetes. These include being overweight or obese, caesarean section and the medical management of neonates who are at increased risk of hypoglycaemia (see Chapter 8). It is therefore important to avoid separation, have early skin-to-skin contact and encourage early feeding. If separation is unavoidable, the mother should be encouraged to express frequently, eight to ten times a day.

To avoid formula milk supplementation, some professionals recommend that mothers with diabetes express colostrum in late pregnancy, freeze it and bring it to hospital in case the newborn baby requires it. East *et al.* (2014) conducted a systematic review to evaluate the benefits and harms of the expression and storage of breastmilk in late pregnancy finding a lack of robust evidence due to the concerns about premature labour. This led to the DAME (Diabetes and Antenatal Milk Expressing) study, a multicentred, unblinded, randomised control trial (Forster *et al.*, 2017). They concluded that there is no harm in advising women with diabetes to express milk twice a day from 36 weeks of gestation if they are at low risk of complications.

Mothers with diabetes who choose to breastfeed return to their pre-pregnancy weights more quickly and have also been found to have more stable blood glucose levels, requiring less insulin than their pre-pregnancy requirement (Stenhouse, 2018).

Practice recommendations: diabetes

- Skin-to-skin contact: As well as encouraging an early breastfeed, this reduces crying and regulates temperature and breathing and thus conserves energy and reduces the risk of hypoglycaemia.
- Avoid maternal and infant separation when possible.
- In response to the delayed lactogenesis, encourage breastfeeding eight to ten times a day or express breastmilk if this is not possible.
- To ensure lactation is adequate, there should be careful assessment of the infant's hydration, wet nappies and changing stool, and signs of jaundice.
- Hypoglycaemia can be a problem for mothers with insulin-dependent diabetes. If the mother's blood glucose is low, she should have a high-sugar snack such as a milkshake or biscuit (Jackson, 2004). It is important to avoid a hypoglycaemic attack when breastfeeding; if it does occur, Jackson (2004) suggests rapid treatment of one of the following: three or four glucose tablets, 150 ml Lucozade or fruit juice, or 200 ml of a fizzy drink followed by a high-carbohydrate food such as bread or cereal.
- If the mother develops cracked nipples, thrush or mastitis, she should treat her diabetes as she would with any other illness and monitor her blood glucose very carefully and alter her insulin as required to avoid hyperglycaemia (Jackson, 2004).

Approximately 525–625 additional calories per day (total, approximately 2,500–2,800 calories per day) are required by a mother during breastfeeding, 200 kcal of which is mobilised from fat stores laid down during pregnancy (Jackson, 2004). It is thought that mothers with type 1 diabetes may require an additional 50 g of carbohydrate per day to ensure adequate lactation. Jackson (2004) recommends that the mother checks her blood glucose before each feed, even at night and eats a snack to prevent hypoglycaemia. The mother must also be made aware that it is normal to feel thirstier during breastfeeding, and by checking her blood glucose level, she should be able to differentiate this thirst from that of the symptoms of hyperglycaemia.

Obesity

The Department of Health & Social Care (2020) states that 63 per cent of adults in England are overweight or obese – 41 per cent of men and 30 per cent of women are overweight, and 26 per cent of men and 29 per cent of women are obese (obesity being defined as having a body mass index [BMI] of 30 kg/m² or over and overweight 25–29.9 kg/m²). Obesity prevalence is associated with deprivation and is a risk factor for type 2 diabetes, cardiovascular disease and a number of other medical conditions.

Women with a booking BMI ≥ 30 require appropriate specialist advice and support antenatally and postnatally regarding the benefits, initiation and maintenance of breastfeeding (RCOG, 2018). They are at greater risk of developing conditions that challenge successful breastfeeding, such as diabetes mellitus, gestational diabetes, postpartum haemorrhage and pre-eclampsia. They are also at greater risk of having caesarean sections, which makes them significantly less likely to breastfeed (Avici *et al.*, 2014; Keely *et al.*, 2015). Infants born to obese mothers are also at risk of pre-term birth, shoulder dystocia, macrosomia and poor APGAR scores and of being admitted to the neonatal unit (Avici *et al.*, 2014). These higher rates of obstetric and neonatal problems associated with obesity increase the risk of separation of the mother and infant.

Furthermore, women with a BMI greater than 29 kg/m² have been associated with delayed lactogenesis II and reduced duration of breastfeeding due to lower levels of prolactin (Rasmussen and Kjolhede, 2004; Turcksin *et al.*, 2013; Preusting *et al.*, 2017). Rasmussen and Kjolhede (2004) suggested that this may be because progesterone is a fat-soluble hormone. In obese women, the rate of clearance of progesterone following birth may be delayed, thus inhibiting the action of prolactin on the lactocytes. Insulin resistance may also contribute to the delay in lactogenesis II, which can be as much as 85.2 hours (Preusting *et al.*, 2017).

Verret-Chalifour *et al.* (2015) reported that obese women are less likely to choose and initiate breastfeeding, and the duration of breastfeeding is shorter. The Office for Health Improvement Disparity (2022b) conducted a cross-sectional ecological study to understand the association at a small area level between breastfeeding prevalence and children's weight status in the early years and also between breastfeeding prevalence and mothers' weight status during subsequent pregnancy. The study concluded that areas with higher levels of breastfeeding tend to have slightly lower proportions of mothers and children living with obesity and overweight, independent of other factors such as deprivation. Areas with high levels of risk factors for obesity and overweight are likely to have higher rates of children and mothers living with obesity and overweight than areas with similar levels of breastfeeding demonstrating the impact of deprivation.

In addition, obese mothers may lack confidence and have poor body image. The problem is further exacerbated by the tendency for obese women to have physical difficulties due to having large heavy breasts, which may contribute to problems with positioning and attachment, resulting in poor milk supply and nipple trauma (Keely *et al.*, 2015). As well as additional support to initiate lactation, donor milk supplementation for the newborn may be considered.

Adsit and Hewlings (2022) conducted a systematic review on the impact of bariatric surgery on breastfeeding. They recognised the need for further research in this area but reported that after bariatric surgery, breastmilk is adequate in nutrients and breastfeeding should be encouraged with monitoring and micronutrient supplementation.

Practice recommendations: obesity

- Encourage skin-to-skin contact.
- Encourage feeding eight to ten times a day until lactogenesis II is established to encourage lactation. Infants of obese mothers have higher levels of plasma insulin and are therefore at risk of hypoglycaemic episodes that could lead to seizures. Regular feeding will alleviate this and avoid the need for supplementation, ensuring the infant is well hydrated and preventing weight loss.
- Avoid maternal–infant separation when possible.
- Positioning the baby at the breast is a challenge, and obese mothers need a lot of encouragement and support. Large, heavy breasts may need support, such as a rolled-up towel, under the breast. Care must be taken if the baby is being fed in the underarm position so that the heavy breasts do not lie on top of the baby.
- Some obese mothers may feel anxious and embarrassed, which has a negative effect on the let-down reflex. It is important therefore to provide emotional support and to provide an environment that is conducive to putting the mother at ease.
- If the mother's nipples are flat, she may need to use a syringe or a breast pump first to pull out the nipples (see Chapter 6).
- Careful hygiene of the skin folds of the breasts is important to avoid itching and infection.

Polycystic ovary syndrome

Polycystic ovary syndrome (PCOS) often starts in adolescence and is a complex syndrome causing ovarian, endocrine and metabolic dysfunction. Ovaries are usually bigger than usual with a large number of small follicles on the outer surface that rarely ovulate. Because a woman with PCOS rarely ovulates, fertility is a major problem. Women with PCOS are also at increased risk obesity, diabetes mellitus and gestational diabetes, which may have an impact on lactogenesis. Biloš (2017) identified a limited evidence base with conflicting results about the success of breastfeeding for women with PCOS and a lack of understanding that PCOS plays in lactation. It is, however, thought that insulin resistance may have a role. Joham *et al.* (2016) conducted a cross-sectional study involving 4,898 women to examine the breastfeeding women with and without PCOS and the relation with BMI and concluded that after adjusting for BMI, PCOS status alone did not appear to be related to breastfeeding initiation and duration. They also highlighted that PCOS drives hyperandrogenism and insulin resistance.

Approximately 10 per cent of the female population is thought to have PCOS, but not all present with health problems and may not know they have it until they have problems with breastfeeding – usually insufficient milk supply. Some mothers with PCOS may also have an overproduction of milk (galactorrhea – see later in this chapter). Either way, mothers with PCOS need a great deal of support and encouragement to commence breastfeeding and to continue.

Practice recommendations: polycystic ovary syndrome

- Encourage skin-to-skin contact.
- Encourage early and frequent feeding with additional milk expression.
- Galactagogues may be required.
- Provide close monitoring of milk transfer and that the infant is thriving.

Postpartum haemorrhage

Postpartum haemorrhage can impede lactogenesis II due to the traumatic nature of the labour and resulting fatigue. The blood loss and hypotension may cause ischaemia to the pituitary gland and inhibit the production of prolactin. In rare cases, this can result in Sheehan's syndrome (necrosis of the pituitary gland), resulting in failure to lactate (Thompson *et al.*, 2010; Henry and Britz, 2013).

In addition to pharmaceutical treatments, postpartum haemorrhage is often managed with nipple stimulation or breastfeeding within 15 minutes of the birth, which leads to the secretion of oxytocin, and the resulting uterine contractions reduce postpartum bleeding (Almutairi, 2021). However, a randomised controlled trial by Abedi *et al.* (2016) stated there was insufficient evidence to evaluate this. Furthermore, Almutairi *et al.* (2020) suggested skin-to-skin contact and breastfeeding may have positive impact on length of third stage of labour and postpartum bleeding but recognised the limitations of their study.

Practice recommendations: postpartum haemorrhage

- Encourage skin-to-skin contact.
- Encourage early and regular breastfeeding.
- Avoid maternal–infant separation.
- Empty the breast by feeding or expressing as frequently as possible in the first two weeks (approximately eight to ten times a day) to maximise milk production capacity.
- Provide continuing support and education, with position and attachment and assessment of breastfeeds.
- Assess milk transfer by close observation of the baby, including weight and nappies for urine and stool (see Chapter 3).
- Early and regular breastfeeding also stimulates the production of oxytocin, which causes uterine contraction and reduces blood loss (Thompson *et al.*, 2010).

Breast surgery and anomalies

Breast anomalies can be congenital or acquired and can cause serious problems for women who would like to breastfeed but because of the lack of confidence find it difficult. Ectopic breasts (mammary heterotopia), or supernumerary breast tissue, is the most common congenital abnormality and can be found anywhere on the milk line from the axilla to pubic region, although 20 per cent occur in the axilla and may lactate following childbirth. These women need extra support to increase their confidence and to learn effective positioning and attachment.

Breast surgery for augmentation or reduction has become one of the most common forms of plastic surgery and is not a contraindication to breastfeeding, but mothers with implants may need additional support. Bompy *et al.* (2019) conducted a survey by telephone of 1,316 women who had breast implants. Of the 75 (7 per cent) women who gave birth after their surgery, 51 wanted to breastfeed (68 per cent). They found that women with implants had a 75 per cent chance of successfully breastfeeding, an 82 per cent probability with retromuscular implants and 17 per cent with retroglandular implants. They found no difference for type of surgery, surgical approach or type of implant. An earlier systematic review (Schiff *et al.*, 2014) that resulted in a review of only three studies to assess breastfeeding outcomes among women with breast implants found no significant difference in initiating breastfeeding, finding that women with implants were 40 per cent less likely to breastfeed.

Breast augmentation is the insertion of either a silicone or saline-filled implant under the pectoralis muscle (submuscular, where the tissue and nerves are relatively undisturbed) or on top of the muscle next to the glandular tissues (subglandular, which may cause greater interference with milk production). The techniques used for inserting the implant are:

- *Transaxillary*: near the axilla but placed below the muscle.
- *Inframammary*: under the breast but placed on top of the muscle next to the glandular tissue, which may cause pressure.
- *Periareolar*: incision around the areola resulting in ductal, glandular and nerve damage; the implant is also inserted above the muscle.

The aim of breast reduction is to remove the volume of breast tissue, which includes both glandular and fatty tissue and which may result in reduced milk-producing ability. There are numerous surgical techniques, but it appears that mothers who are more likely to breastfeed successfully have had surgery that does not completely sever the areola and nipple but instead moves them while still being attached to the 'pedicle', ducts, nerves and blood supply. Many women have reduced nipple sensation following the procedure, which may negatively affect the let-down reflex. Some mothers may also complain of oversensitivity during the healing process. Bearing in mind that some women may only have nine main ducts (Ramsay *et al.*, 2005), removal of any of these is likely to cause a reduction in milk supply.

Some mothers with breast anomalies, or following breast surgery, report production of colostrum but do not go on to lactate fully. Therefore, careful observation of the infant is required to ensure there is effective milk production and transfer and that the infant is thriving. It must also be remembered that the mother may have had surgery for poorly developed breasts, which may have been a consequence of polycystic ovaries.

> **Practice recommendations: breast surgery and anomalies**
>
> - Establish a good history regarding the breast problem or type of surgery.
> - Encourage skin-to-skin contact.
> - Encourage early and regular breastfeeding.
> - Avoid maternal–infant separation.
> - Empty the breast by feeding or expressing as frequently as possible in the first two weeks (approximately eight to ten times a day) to maximise milk production capacity.
> - Provide continuing support with position and attachment and assessment of breastfeeds.
> - Assess milk transfer by close observation of the baby: weight and nappies for urine and stool (see Chapter 3).

Epilepsy

Mothers with epilepsy and taking antiepileptic drugs should be encouraged to breastfeed, but they should be taught to recognise any signs of toxicity or side effects (NICE, 2022b). Breastfeeding may reduce withdrawal symptoms in the newborn, such as hyperirritability and poor sucking. However, some drugs may have side effects that may cause the infant to be sleepy and lead to difficulties with maintaining attachment. Infants should be monitored for sedation, feeding problems, weight gain and developmental milestones and referred for medical advice if there any concerns.

It is also important for the mother to consider where she feeds her infant so that, if she does have a seizure, the risk of an accident is minimised. It is advisable to sit on the floor or an area where the infant will not fall.

Hyperlactation or galactorrhea

Hyperlactation is the overproduction of breastmilk and is most commonly caused by breastfeeding mismanagement, medications or hyperprolactinaemia. The mother will have a constant feeling of fullness and may leak or spray copious amounts of milk from the other breast during feeding, and she will leak in between feeds. Because the breasts are always full, she is at higher risk of mastitis and developing an abscess. Livingstone (1996) suggested that problems are most likely to occur when the mother switches her infant from one breast to the other before the first has been effectively emptied and the infant has had a chance to receive the high-fat milk or because of poor position and attachment.

Hyperlactation may also pose problems for the infant during a feed as she or he struggles to cope with the flow of the feed, possibly resulting in breast refusal. Also, the infant may be unable to empty the breast adequately to get the high-fat milk, which will result in poor weight gain and failure to thrive. The infant will also present with colic and explosive, watery, green stools (Figure 7.1).

Twins

Mothers of multiple births can successfully breastfeed and should be encouraged and supported to do so. It is the role of the healthcare professional to instil confidence in a

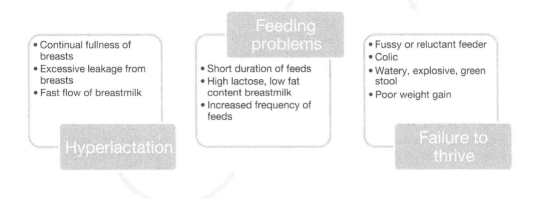

- Continual fullness of breasts
- Excessive leakage from breasts
- Fast flow of breastmilk

Hyperlactation

Feeding problems

- Short duration of feeds
- High lactose, low fat content breastmilk
- Increased frequency of feeds

- Fussy or reluctant feeder
- Colic
- Watery, explosive, green stool
- Poor weight gain

Failure to thrive

Figure 7.1 The consequences of hyperlactation

mother's ability to breastfeed. Informing her of any support groups during pregnancy may help with this so that she can see other mothers of twins breastfeeding. The main challenges the mother faces are prematurity (see Chapter 8), tiredness and time. Twins can be fed separately or simultaneously; however, it is advisable to encourage mothers to

---

Practice recommendations: hyperlactation

There is limited evidence available regarding the management of hyperlactation, and recommendations are mainly anecdotal (Trimeloni and Spencer, 2016); however, the aim is to improve milk removal and drainage in each breast. Treatment is complex and is not achieved by reducing the frequency of breastfeeding but by instead restricting feeds to one breast only to allow a reduction of milk supply to occur through the build-up of the FIL in the other breast. By feeding at one breast only, the infant is more likely to drain the breast effectively, receiving the fattier milk, which will be more satisfying and thus increase time intervals between feeds. There is an increased risk of blocked ducts and mastitis, and therefore this management requires careful monitoring.

Another suggestion is *block feeding*, whereby the infant is offered the same breast for a block period of time during the day and has several consecutive feeds at this breast before doing the same on the other (van Veldhuizen-Staas, 2007, Eglash, 2014). Van Veldhuizen-Staas (2007) recommends full drainage and block feeding. This starts with, as near as possible, complete drainage of both breasts using a mechanical breast pump. The infant is then offered the breasts where they will receive high-fat milk. She suggests that this may have been the first time these infants will have had high-fat milk, and they will be satiated and sleep following the feed. The rest of the day is split into blocks of time starting with three hours. As the infant demands a feed, the same breast is offered for that block of time. At the end of this block of time, the infant is offered the other breast for all the demanded feeds in the next block of time. The time blocks should be individually assessed depending on the individual symptoms.

Herbal remedies, such as sage and peppermint tea, jasmine flowers (topically) and parsley, are also thought to reduce milk supply (Eglash, 2014).

breastfeed both infants together, as soon as they are feeding effectively, to reduce the time feeding takes and to establish an adequate milk supply.

The most common position for feeding is the underarm hold, but any position the mother can manage that adheres to the principles of positioning and attachment will work. Some mothers find a V-shaped pillow useful to support infants when feeding them simultaneously in the early days, but care must be taken that it does not interfere with positioning and attachment (Figure 7.2).

Tiredness is a common complaint, and family and friends often ask to help by feeding the twins. It would be more helpful if they helped with family chores such as cooking, cleaning, washing and ironing or looking after other children to allow the mother time to rest and spend with her twins to establish breastfeeding.

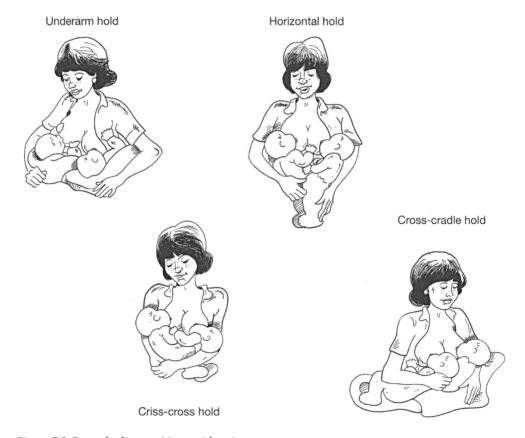

Figure 7.2 Breastfeeding positions with twins

Concluding comments

HIV is the only condition for which it is recommended that breastfeeding be avoided. However, there are a number of conditions or situations with which breastfeeding may need to be temporarily avoided or may compromise the initiation, duration and exclusivity of breastfeeding. This chapter has described some of the situations healthcare professionals may come into contact with in clinical practice, but it is by no means exhaustive.

Although many of these conditions or situations have individual complexities, it is clear that the principles of establishing and maintaining an adequate milk supply are very similar. In all cases, it is important that a breastfeeding assessment is made followed by observation of a full breastfeed to check position and attachment and milk transfer. Breastfeeding straight after birth is crucial, when possible, followed by regular stimulation of the breast by the infant or expressing by hand or with a pump. Skin-to-skin contact should also be recommended at all ages. Ongoing support by knowledgeable healthcare practitioners is essential for mothers in challenging situations.

Scenario 1

Harry is four days old. He was 4.2 kg at birth. After a 15-hour labour, Harry was delivered by caesarean section for 'failure to progress'. His mother, Stacey, had gestational diabetes, sustained a 1,200-ml postpartum haemorrhage and was transfused two units of packed red blood.

Skin-to-skin was brief following birth, and Harry was reluctant to suck for the first couple of days and had some cup feeds. Stacey is tired and doesn't think she has enough milk to feed him and is thinking about bottle feeding. Stacey now has sore nipples. Yesterday he weighed 3.7 kg, and the paediatrician requested that he be weighed again today. Today he is 3.6 kg.

What would you do?

Scenario 2

Andrea has been successfully breastfeeding Eric but has been invited for her COVID-19 booster vaccination and has been told by a family member that if she has it, she will have to stop breastfeeding. She wants to continue breastfeeding and ask you what she should do.

What advice will you give Andrea?

Further reading

- WHO (2016) *Guideline Updates on HIV and Breastfeeding. The Duration of Breastfeeding and Support from Health Services to Improve Feeding Practices Among Mothers Living with HIV*, Geneva: WHO.
- WHO/UNICEF (2009) *Acceptable Medical Reasons for the Use of Breast-milk Substitutes*, Geneva: WHO.

Resources

- COVID-19
  www.nhs.uk/pregnancy/keeping-well/pregnancy-breastfeeding-fertility-and-cor-
  onavirus-covid-19-vaccination
  www.rcog.org.uk/guidance/coronavirus-covid-19-pregnancy-and-women-s-
  health/vaccination/covid-19-vaccines-pregnancy-and-breastfeeding-faqs/

- Breastfeeding Network
  www.breastfeedingnetwork.org.uk/detailed-information/drugs-in-breastmilk

- Le Leche League
  www.llli.org/breastfeeding-info/

- Twins Trust
  https://twinstrust.org/

- Multiple Births Foundation
  www.multiplebirths.org.uk

- NHS HIV and AIDS
  www.nhs.uk/conditions/hiv-and-aids

- NICE BNF- Epilepsy
  https://bnf.nice.org.uk/treatment-summaries/epilepsy

8 Infants with special needs

Breastmilk should be the first choice of infant nutrition for infants separated from their mothers and for those with special needs. Exclusive breastfeeding should be protected, with no other food or drugs being given, unless medically indicated, because of the benefits breastmilk confers on both mother and infant (WHO, 2021a).

Infants with special needs, such as low birth weight and prematurity, are at higher risk of poor outcomes following birth, throughout childhood and on to adulthood (Katz *et al.*, 2013). A high proportion of infants from this category are also from disadvantaged socio-economic backgrounds (Moser *et al.*, 2003). In neonatal units, parents are encouraged to provide breastmilk for their infants as part of the care package, and this presents a great opportunity for healthcare professionals to promote breastfeeding.

There will be situations when breastmilk substitutes will be required; however, these should be medically indicated, and clear protocols should be developed to deal with these situations. The WHO and UNICEF (2009, p. 7) published a list of acceptable medical reasons for temporary or long-term use of breastmilk substitutes:

- **Infants who should not receive breastmilk or any other milk except specialised formula:**

DOI: 10.4324/9781003282341-8

- *Infants with galactosaemia*:

  This is a rare genetic trait incompatible with breastfeeding. Symptoms include vomiting, jaundice, hepatosplenomegaly and bleeding. Without treatment, galactose builds up and can cause kidney, liver, nerve and eye damage. All milk products should be removed from the infant's diet and replaced a special galactose-free formula is needed (IMD Scotland, 2017).

- *Infants with maple syrup urine disease*:

  This is an aminoacidopathy and presents with poor feeding and weight gain, vomiting, seizures and lethargy. Breastfeeding may delay onset of these symptoms. Breastfeeding is possible, but infants require careful monitoring and supplementation with a special formula free of leucine, isoleucine and valine (Frazier *et al.*, 2014; IMD Scotland, 2017).

- *Infants with phenylketonuria*:

  A special phenylalanine-free formula is needed. However, breastmilk has lower levels of phenylalanine than formula milk and, combined with a phenylalanine-free formula, close monitoring and expert support and advice, breastfeeding is possible (Banta-Wright *et al.*, 2012; IMD Scotland, 2017).

- **Infants may need other food in addition to breastmilk for a limited period if they are:**

  - born weighing less than 1,500 g;
  - born at less than 32 weeks' gestational age; or
  - at risk of hypoglycaemia (preterm, small for gestational age, have suffered a hypoxic episode, are ill infants or infants whose mothers have diabetes, with low blood sugar levels).

This chapter focuses on the issues related to infants with special needs and some other conditions or situations, such as poor weight gain, hypernatraemia and tongue-tie, which may also pose problems and challenges with breastfeeding.

Learning outcomes

By the end of this chapter, you will be able to:

- identify conditions or situations with which breastfeeding may be temporarily challenged and
- provide evidence-based information for mothers to help them maintain lactation when their infants are unwell or if they are separated.

Mapping to UNICEF Baby Friendly Initiative (BFI) Education learning outcomes (2019a)
  By the end of the programme, students will:

Theme		Learning outcomes
Theme 4: Manage the challenges	11.	Be able to apply their knowledge of the physiology of lactation and infant feeding to support effective management of challenges which may arise at any time during breastfeeding.
	12.	Have an understanding of the special circumstances which can affect lactation and breastfeeding (e.g. when mother and baby are separated, including preterm and sick infants) and be able to support mothers to overcome the challenge.

Strategies for care in the neonatal unit

UNICEF UK BFI (2022) developed a set of evidence-based standards with the aim of transforming neonatal units and improving outcomes for vulnerable infants. Neonatal units can apply for accreditation (see Appendix 3 for further detail).

Parents should be provided with evidence-based information about the short- and long-term benefits of breastmilk for infants with special needs so they can make an informed decision about their choice of infant feeding. However, the principles of supporting breastfeeding for these infants are the same as for healthy term infants:

- Early feeding following birth (when clinically appropriate).
- Skin-to-skin contact.
- Correct position and attachment.
- If the infant is unable to suckle, breastmilk should be expressed and given by an alternative method that will not interfere with future breastfeeding.

Assessing readiness to feed should be based on:

- gestational age;
- physiological status and alertness;
- sucking pattern; and
- feeding cues.

                                        (McGrath and Braescu, 2004; Shaker, 2013)

If an infant is unable to breastfeed or requires alternative methods of infant feeding, this should be discussed with the parents and their decision recorded in the care plan. As with term infants, teats should be avoided in case 'nipple confusion' develops (Zimmerman and Thompson, 2015). A more suitable method of providing nutrition should be used that will not interfere with future feeding at the breast. McInnes and Chambers (2008a) conducted a systematic review of 27 papers to identify interventions to promote breastfeeding or breastmilk feeding for infants admitted to the neonatal unit. The only conclusive interventions that appear to support breastfeeding they could find were skin-to-skin contact, postnatal support and the use of galactagogues. They concluded that there was a lack of research into interventions such as cup feeding and that neonatal unit staff needed to work with individual mothers and infants to determine the most appropriate plan of care. They did, however, highlight that, given the evidence to support the physical and emotional benefits of breastfeeding for the mother–infant dyad, these plans should support mothers to express breastmilk and breastfeed to maximise milk production, increase maternal confidence and promote continued breastfeeding following discharge.

Expressing breastmilk

Most normal healthy infants demand 8–12 feeds per day within the first 24–48 hours with gaps no longer than four hours during the day and six hours at night. Mothers should be encouraged to express breastmilk as soon as possible after birth to stimulate the production of prolactin to prime the lactocytes to establish milk production, as well as provide colostrum for the infant, ideally within the first two hours. The aim is to establish a milk supply of approximately 750 ml/day by day 10. Emphasis should be on frequent expressing and the avoidance of long intervals between expressions.

Chapter 4 explains the technique for hand expression and the use of mechanical breast pumps. Hand expression is useful for expressing small quantities of colostrum that can be collected in a syringe. Because mothers of ill infants may spend a lot of time in the neonatal unit, it is important to provide a supportive environment, physical and psychological, and to provide facilities that are comfortable for expressing milk and privacy if preferred. Once discharged from hospital, mothers express their breastmilk at home and need clear guidelines about the safe handling, storage and transport of the breastmilk. There should also be a system for the provision of breast pumps for home use while the mother and infant are separated.

UNICEF UK BFI neonatal standards (2022, pp. 10–13) recommend the following to enable babies to receive breastmilk and to breastfeed when possible.

- Mothers are enabled to express milk as soon as possible, ideally within the first two hours.
- Mothers learn how to express effectively by hand and pump (as appropriate to individual need) and learn how to store milk.
- Mothers are supported to express frequently to optimise supply, especially in first two to three weeks.
- Mothers have access to adequate and effective expressing equipment to use on the unit and at home.
- A formal review of expressing takes place a minimum of four times in the first two weeks and there is access to further help with expressing if milk supplies are inadequate or less than 750 mls by day 10.
- Expressing is frequently checked, on an informal basis, after the first two weeks.
- The unit has an environment conducive to expressing.

Activity

Do you provide 'colostrum packs' in your unit? These ready-made packs contain the equipment and information to encourage mothers to express colostrum that can be saved or used immediately.

'Double pumping' or simultaneous pumping is encouraged as it saves time and increases prolactin levels and therefore milk production (Renfrew *et al.*, 2009; Mansoori and Salmani, 2020). Both breasts are pumped using a mechanical breast pump for about 10–15 minutes, whereas for single pumping it can take approximately 15 minutes at each breast. Breast massage prior to pumping may increase expressed milk volumes (McInnes and Chambers, 2006). However, McInnes and Chambers (2006) reported that some mothers preferred a hand pump to an electrical pump.

Mothers should be instructed to store the required quantity of breastmilk for each feed in a separate sterile container with her name, date, time of expression and unique identifying number. If not used immediately, breastmilk should be stored in a fridge designated for this purpose only. Temperature recordings should be taken daily and should not exceed 2–4°C. Expressed breastmilk should be used within 24 hours or frozen in a freezer at a temperature of –20°C for a maximum of three months. If the mother expresses at home, she should follow the same guidelines and transport the breastmilk in an insulated container with ice packs to the neonatal unit.

Activity

What is the local policy for the safe handling, storage and transport of the breast-milk in your neonatal unit?

Skin-to-skin or kangaroo care

Kangaroo care gets its name from the marsupial, the kangaroo, which births its infants at an early gestation and then incubates them by carrying them in a pouch. Kangaroo care was developed in Colombia in response to inadequate resources for ill infants (Charpak *et al.*, 2005). Instead of having the preterm infant cared for in an incubator, the infant is cared for next to the skin of the mother or father for a prolonged period of time. The infant is placed skin to skin (usually only wearing a nappy and possibly a hat) in an upright position between the mother's breasts or on the father's chest.

Infants who are separated from their mothers have increased heart rate and blood pressure and higher levels of cortisol. The touch and warmth of skin contact reduce these symptoms and increase oxytocin levels in infants, which has an analgesic effect. Not only does kangaroo care have a soothing effect on preterm infants by providing comfort, physiological stability and improved sleep, but it also encourages bonding, parenting behaviour (Johnston *et al.*, 2008; Bergman, 2019) and increased breastfeeding by providing easier access to find the breast and attach, allowing the mother to learn feeding cues (McInnes and Chambers, 2008a). Even if the infant is unable to suckle, kangaroo care enables the infant to learn to recognise the smell of the mother's skin.

Bergman *et al.* (2004) conducted a randomised controlled trial and found that infants weighing 1,200–2,199 g who had skin-to-skin contact were more able to maintain their temperature after six hours than those in an incubator. A systematic review conducted by Conde-Agudelo and Díaz-Rossello (2016) supported these findings and found that kangaroo care reduced mortality rate, severe illness, infection and respiratory problems and was related to an increase in weight, length and breastfeeding duration. They also recommended further research in this area of practice. Roller (2005) reported mothers describing kangaroo care as a calming and positive experience for them as well.

The UNICEF UK BFI neonatal standards (2022) recommend:

- Skin contact is used to induce instinctive feeding behaviours.
- Staff are educated to understand the value of skin contact for encouraging breastfeeding.
- Privacy is provided in an unhurried environment for mothers as they learn to breastfeed.

It is important that parents are informed about the benefits of skin-to-skin contact, doing it as often as possible, in an unhurried environment as soon as the infant's condition allows. Renfrew *et al.* (2009) found that short periods of skin-to-skin contact of up to an hour, at all visits, increased the duration of breastfeeding.

Galactagogues

Some mothers may have difficulty in establishing and maintaining lactation, and in addition to skin-to-skin contact and frequently expressing milk, they may need galactagogues such as domperidone or metoclopramide. Renfrew *et al.* (2009) suggested that this line of treatment is more useful for mothers whose lactation is not meeting the infant's needs rather than for those who have recently given birth. Galactagogues increase prolactin levels by blocking dopamine, which acts as prolactin inhibitor. Unfortunately, they are not licensed to augment lactation, and there is a lack of evidence to support dosage. However, the most common prescribed is domperidone 10 mg, taken orally three times a day for up to a week (BFN, 2019d). If this does not work, the dose can be continued or increased (see local guidelines), whilst monitoring for any adverse side effects. In a secondary analysis for the EMPOWER trial, Asztalos *et al.* (2019) concluded that after the first week following lactation support, such as expression, where breastmilk volumes were still low, domperidone may be offered to augment production. Once lactation is established, the drug can be withdrawn slowly. Anecdotally, two or three capsules a day of fenugreek may also help improve milk supply, but this should be taken in consultation with a doctor as it can interfere with the action of other medications. Other natural remedies include anise, basil, blessed thistle, caraway, chasteberry and fennel. In 2020, Foong *et al.* published a systematic review of oral galactagogues but found limited evidence to support their use.

Preterm infants

BLISS estimate approximately one in 13 infants are born preterm (less than 37 weeks' gestation) in the UK every year. Breastfeeding preterm infants can be particularly challenging for mothers and healthcare professionals supporting them, as the infants' needs vary according to their size, gestation and physiological stability. Preterm infants have immature gastrointestinal tracts with increased permeability and susceptibility to infection. Breastmilk has high levels of anti-infective properties and prebiotics (good bacteria), which reduce the incidence of necrotising enterocolitis, diarrhoea, respiratory infection and the development of allergies (see Chapter 1). Breastmilk is also more readily digested than formula and has a low renal solute load. Some infants may require prescribed formula fortification of the breastmilk or supplementation if the volumes of expressed breastmilk are insufficient or donor milk is unavailable.

Lactogenesis II is significantly delayed in mothers of extremely premature infants for a number of reasons, such as incomplete mammary growth, the stress and anxiety that mothers of preterm infants face and delay in breastfeeding or initiation of expressing breastmilk. Henderson *et al.* (2008) suggested that lactation can be further reduced in those treated with corticosteroids (betamethasone) in the antenatal period between 28 and 34 weeks' gestation, when birth occurs three to nine days later. This is further compounded if mothers do not express milk more than six times a day. Riddle and Nommsen-Rivers (2016) reported that mothers with low milk supply were more likely to have had diabetes in pregnancy compared with those with other lactation difficulties. Hartmann and Ramsay (2006) suggest that the shorter length of pregnancy and poor placental function, resulting in a reduction in placental lactogen levels, may make the situation worse.

These problems are also compounded by the fact that preterm infants:

- may have a poor or absent suck-swallow-breathe coordination (dependent on gestational age);
- lack 'cheek pads', leading to a weak suck;
- may have nasal prongs, feeding tubes and so on, leading to a poor oral experience;
- may have lung disease or other impairments of a physical or neurological nature;
- may lack the energy to complete a feed; or
- require medically indicated supplementary feeds.

It is therefore imperative that there is a supportive and positive developmental environment that is private, warm and quiet, with reduced light and noise levels, to encourage skin-to-skin contact or kangaroo care. Skin-to-skin or kangaroo care is an important aspect of care for premature infants; not only does it help regulate breathing, heart rate and temperature, but it also enhances milk ejection and access to the breast for the infant (Moore *et al.*, 2012). In a randomised controlled trial, Hake-Brooks and Anderson (2008) found that preterm infants, 32–36 weeks, who had unlimited kangaroo care, breastfed for longer than infants in the control group who received traditional nursery care (5.08 months as opposed to 2.05 months). Parker *et al.* (2012) found in a pilot study that milk expression within one hour after birth was effective in decreasing the time to lactogenesis II and increasing milk supply in the first week.

Interventions may be introduced into neonatal units to encourage preterm infants to suckle. Non-nutritive sucking using dummies or at the breast may be used in neonatal units to provide comfort, to encourage a sucking technique and to provide a positive oral experience (Harding, 2009; Foster *et al.*, 2016). However, dummies are withdrawn by approximately 32–34 weeks to encourage breastfeeding. Nipple shields may also be used to make it easier for the infant to latch on to the breast. Aloysius and Lozano (2007) conducted a study of 12 mothers, over a one-year period, whose infants were in the neonatal unit and who requested a nipple shield. The reasons for using nipple shields were flat or inverted nipples or the infant's being used to a firmer teat. The mothers reported that the shields helped with attachment; however, one discontinued using the shield because she believed it reduced her milk supply and went on to successfully breastfeed. The study concluded that some preterm infants may benefit from the use of nipple shields in the transition period to breastfeeding from tube or bottle feeding and that it may in fact increase milk yield. Further research is required in this area.

Depending on the infant's physical condition and gestation, infants who are unable to suckle at the breast can be given expressed breastmilk by alternative methods such as a nasogastric tube, syringe or cup (see Chapter 9).

Between 30 and 34 weeks, preterm infants are able to lap milk from a cup, which gives the advantage of providing satisfying oral experience and gastric stimulation. With cup feeding, the infant is able to control the amount and rate of the feed similar to breastfeeding. Therefore, the intake for preterm infants should be monitored over a 24-hour period rather than forcing the calculated amount at each feed. Preterm infants who are cup fed have higher oxygen saturation levels and are less likely to desaturate during a feed, and they have lower heart rates (Penny *et al.*, 2018).

By 36 weeks' gestation, infants should be able to coordinate the suck-swallow-breathe reflex to feed at the breast (McGrath and Braescu, 2004) but may lack energy to sustain a full feed; in these circumstances, the infant may benefit from 'switch nursing'. Switch nursing or feeding is when the infant is switched from one breast to the other two or three times during each feed as the infant's sucking slows down and swallowing is less frequent. This enables the infant to get the high-calorie milk following a let-down reflex to increase the infant's energy to enable him or her to feed for longer and go on to demand feed. There is concern, however, that the infant does not feed long enough to get the high-fat breastmilk because he or she may not empty the breast, and switch nursing is therefore only to be used as a temporary measure. Infants who are born small for gestational age are usually very hungry and feed frequently and regularly. Despite this, they may still require breastfeeds to be supplemented to meet their nutritional needs.

Hypoxic infants

Hypoxia can occur at any gestation, either because of an in utero event or at birth. It is usually caused by placental insufficiency, cord issues or other problems such as meconium aspiration. In these circumstances, the commencement of enteral feeding may be delayed and replaced with intravenous nutrition because of concerns regarding gut ischaemia and injury, but this remains an area of debate (Young *et al.*, 2011). Breastmilk is particularly valuable for infants following a hypoxic event, when the motility of the gastrointestinal tract may have been affected, as it is more easily digested and absorbed while offering anti-infective properties unavailable in formula milk.

As soon as possible after birth, the mother should be encouraged to express colostrum, which can be stored for her infant until required; this will also initiate lactation. When possible, skin-to-skin contact should be promoted. When the infant is able to feed at the breast, the mother will need skilled support, as these infants often have poor suck-swallow-breathe coordination. Supplementation will be required, and a suitable method of administering this should be chosen, avoiding a bottle and teat as these infants are more prone to nipple confusion. Kruger *et al.* (2019) suggested oropharyngeal dysphagia was identified in the majority of infants with hypoxic-ischemic encephalopathy. Hersh *et al.* (2022) suggested when there is a risk of aspiration due to dysphagia, there is a paucity of evidence for the management of breastfeeding with some recommending discontinuing breastfeeding, thickening breastmilk given by bottle or feeding tube.

Jaundice

Neonatal jaundice is extremely common, affecting around 60 per cent of term and 80 per cent of preterm infants in the first week of life and approximately 10 per cent at one month (NICE, 2016). Jaundice can be a very complex problem, and it is essential that midwives can differentiate between physiological jaundice, breastmilk jaundice and jaundice with a pathological cause. In utero fetuses have high levels of fetal red blood cells, which are no longer required following birth and need to be broken down. The haem component of the red blood cells is converted to biliverdin and bilirubin. Some bilirubin is bound to albumin in the circulation, where it is transported to the liver and conjugated. It is then transported via the bile duct to the intestine to be eliminated in the stool. However, some of this bilirubin is reabsorbed into the blood via the enterohepatic circulation and returned to liver for processing. Jaundice is increased in preterm infants due to polycythaemia, following trauma or bruising (forceps or vacuum delivery), infection, metabolic disorders and ineffective feeding.

There are three types of jaundice that midwives must be aware of and able to diagnose to ensure the correct treatment is initiated: pathological jaundice, physiological jaundice and breastmilk jaundice.

Pathological jaundice presents within 24 hours of birth and is the result of an underlying disease such as haemolytic disease or sepsis. It is essential for these infants to have a paediatric review.

Physiological jaundice is more common and is thought to occur in about 50–60 per cent of infants. It usually presents around the third day following birth, fading gradually over the following ten days. It is also more common in breastfed infants. Physiological jaundice is caused by:

- Red blood cell breakdown, leading to increased bilirubin levels and reabsorption
- Reduced albumin levels, reducing the albumin-binding capacity of conjugated bilirubin
- Limited production of glucuronyl transferase to metabolise fat-soluble unconjugated bilirubin to water-soluble conjugated bilirubin
- Enteric reabsorption of unconjugated bilirubin due to delayed clearance of meconium

Serum bilirubin levels should be taken if the jaundice is significant or the infant appears unwell. If the serum bilirubin level is raised (see the threshold table and care pathways in NICE, 2016) or the infant is unwell, the infant should have an urgent medical review and possible treatment with phototherapy or, in extreme cases, blood exchange transfusion. High serum bilirubin levels can be neurotoxic and lead to kernicterus (a form of brain damage) (Levene *et al.*, 2008; NICE, 2016).

Breastfeeding has been associated with physiological jaundice; however, NICE (2016) indicates this is not a reason for discontinuing breastfeeding and suggests it may be due to inadequate support resulting in reduced intake and delay in meconium evacuation. Renfrew *et al.* (2000) identified unrestricted feeds, no supplements and rooming-in as effective treatments.

Practice recommendations: jaundice

- Encourage skin-to-skin contact and rooming-in so the mother can pick up infant feeding cues.
- Encourage regular breastfeeds, at no more than three-hourly intervals, to increase bowel motility, clear meconium and reduce the reabsorption of unconjugated bilirubin. Colostrum acts as a laxative, which purges the bowel of bilirubin. If the infant is sleepy, she or he will need to be wakened.
- Observe and assess breastfeeds to ensure adequate milk transfer.
- If the infant has difficulty feeding, weight loss is more than 7 per cent of the birth weight or there are signs of dehydration, the mother should be encouraged to express breastmilk following the feed and give this as a supplement or 'top-up' via a cup or other appropriate alternative feeding method.
- Infants with jaundice should not be routinely supplemented with formula, dextrose and water.

Physiological jaundice can become worse if the infant does not feed frequently. This is further exacerbated by the fact that jaundiced infants tend to be sleepy and reluctant to feed. Mothers need a lot of support with sleepy infants; unlimited skin-to-skin contact for easy access to the breast should be encouraged to facilitate rooting behaviour and prolactin surges for the maintenance of milk production. Regular breastmilk expression should also be encouraged and given to the infant by cup or spoon.

Prolonged or *breastmilk jaundice* is an unconjugated hyperbilirubinaemia and develops at·four to seven days after birth and lasts for several months; its cause is unknown (Rosenthal, 2014). The infant is asymptomatic, and this condition is rarely of concern; however, other causes should be excluded before coming to this diagnosis (Levene *et al.*, 2008; NICE, 2016).

Hypoglycaemia

Immediately following birth, infants lose their constant glucose supply from their mothers and have to maintain its own plasma glucose levels as well as adapt to intermittent nutrition episodes. Blood glucose levels are maintained by insulin and glucagon levels secreted by the islets of Langerhans in the pancreas. In normal healthy term infants, blood glucose levels drop to approximately 2–2.6 mmol/l (see local protocol) following birth but gradually rise to approximately 3.6 mmol/l after about six hours. Correspondingly, plasma insulin levels decrease following birth, making it more difficult for glucose to be taken up by the cells. In response, glucose serum glucagon levels rise, converting intracellular glycogen stores to glucose (glycogenolysis). The high levels of glucose lead to increased levels of insulin and decreased glucagon levels, but the stores of glycogen decrease rapidly over the first 24 hours after birth. Newborns also have the ability to mobilise alternative fuels through lipolysis and ketogenesis. This is a normal physiological process, and therefore there is no reason to monitor blood glucose levels for normal healthy term infants within the first two to four hours as it will only encourage unnecessary intervention.

Glucose is essential for brain function, and some infants are at risk of hypoglycaemia (plasma glucose less than 2.6 mmol/l) (Levene *et al.*, 2008; Dixon *et al.*, 2017), such as preterm infants; infants who are small or large for gestational age; if there has been birth trauma or hypoxia, infection or hypothermia; infants of mothers with diabetes, and infants of mothers on beta-blockers in the third trimester or at the time of giving birth (causing hyperinsulinaemia) (see Chapter 7 for management of infants of mothers with diabetes). These infants must be identified and correctly managed. Signs of hypoglycaemia include lethargy, tachypnoea or apnoea, hypotonia, irritability, unstable temperature, twitching, convulsions or coma. Jitteriness is not an absolute sign of hypoglycaemia as many infants respond like this to handling in the first few days.

Practice recommendations: high-risk newborns

The following recommendations are based on BAPM (2017) guidance. The main aim is to avoid hypoglycaemia, first by identifying a 'high-risk' infant and then by providing the appropriate care:

- Encourage skin-to-skin contact whenever possible to encourage breastfeeding and maintain body temperature. Avoiding the infant's becoming cold is probably one of the main interventions to prevent hypoglycaemia; ensure the infant is dried and a hat put on. Skin-to-skin contact also stabilises the heart and respiratory rate and reduces crying (Moore *et al.*, 2012). All of this avoids the infant's using up his or her glucagon stores too quickly.

- Encourage an early breastfeed within the first hour following birth, providing support and assessment of attachment.
- Breastfeed in response to feeding cues but no less than three hours apart until blood glucose measurements have been above 2.0 mmol/l on two consecutive occasions. Breastmilk is thought to improve mobilisation of alternative energy sources.
- The first blood glucose should be taken 2–4 hours following birth, before the second feed or when there are clinical signs of hypoglycaemia.
- If the infant is not feeding effectively, continue skin-to-skin contact and teach the mother to express colostrum, which should be given to the infant immediately via a cup, syringe or nasogastric tube (see Chapter 9). Continue this eight to ten times in 24 hours or until breastfeeding is effective. If no breastmilk is available, formula milk can be given at the rate of 10–15 ml/kg, preferably by cup, until colostrum is available. Some infants may require intravenous infusions.

See the BAPM Framework for Practice (2017) for further guidance and pathways.

Postmature infants

Postmature infants have remained in utero as the placental function decreases. They usually have diminished subcutaneous fat and dry and peeling skin. As well as losing subcutaneous fat, postmature infants have begun to lose glycogen stores and may be hypoglycaemic at birth. Maintaining temperature may be a problem, and therefore an early breastfeed and skin-to-skin contact are required to maintain temperature and blood glucose levels (Noble and Rosen-Carole, 2022). Due to their lack of glycogen stores, hypoglycaemia may continue to be a problem, and therefore blood glucose monitoring may be required. Once established, breastfeeding should not be a problem.

Tongue-tie (ankyloglossia)

Tongue-tie, or ankyloglossia, is when the frenulum (membrane), which holds the tongue in place at the floor of the mouth, is either thicker or shorter than normal and is graded level 1–4, with grade 1 being most severe (Trotter, 2010). When the infant cries, the tongue remains fixed to the bottom of the mouth. The tongue has an important role in breastfeeding by positioning the breast in the mouth and creating a vacuum to draw the milk from the breast. Some infants with tongue-tie can breastfeed successfully; however, others may have difficulty attaching to the breast because they cannot open the mouth wide enough to scoop the breast, as the tongue is unable to extend beyond the gum, which in turn affects the tongue's movements when sucking (this can also be a problem for bottle-fed infants.). This means that milk may not be effectively removed from the breast, and the infant 'nipple feeds', which will ultimately cause reduced milk supply, nipple damage, pain and an unsatisfied and hungry infant. Blocked ducts, mastitis and abscesses may all be a result of ineffective milk removal. The infant may also go on to have poor weight gain and growth as well as prolonged jaundice and may be introduced to formula milk (Finigan, 2009). Tongue-tie should be noted at the routine examination of the newborn and a plan of care developed to include additional support with position and attachment and, in some cases, surgery.

Geddes *et al.* (2008) conducted a study to identify whether frenotomy was an effective treatment for tongue-tie. She used ultrasound imaging before and after surgery to assess the infant's tongue action, milk transfer and milk intake. She found that all measures were improved. However, she recommended that cases be individually assessed prior to treatment. Furthermore, NICE (2011) conducted a review of the 2005 guidance and found the procedure to be effective in facilitating breastfeeding for 70 per cent of infants in the review period. Parents' responses were reported to be 'overwhelmingly positive' even if breastfeeding did not continue. However, Cawse-Lucas *et al.* (2015) found no evidence to support frenotomy for improving attachment but identified a 10 per cent improvement in maternal comfort. This was supported by O'Shea *et al.* (2017), who conducted a systematic review. In cases in which breastfeeding is a problem, surgically dividing the tongue-tie may be required (Hogan *et al.*, 2005).

Frenotomy is a quick procedure that, in many cases, does not need a general anaesthetic, but a local anaesthetic is sometimes used. The infant is wrapped up, and the tongue-tie divided with sterile blunt-ended scissors. The mother is given back the infant immediately following the procedure for a feed. The parents should be advised that there will be a few spots of blood only and sometimes a white patch under the tongue that resolves within 48 hours. There is a list of hospitals and contact details where frenotomy is carried out in the UK on the BFI website (www.babyfriendly.org.uk). Some tongue-ties resolve themselves; however, as these infant grow older, they may present problems with weaning and possibly speech.

Weight loss or poor weight gain

Weight loss is normal in the early days of life, related to body fluid adjustments. It usually stops at three to four days and returns to birth weight by three weeks (NICE, 2017). However, continuing weight loss or failure to gain weight can be an indication of either inadequate milk transfer or underlying illness. If the problem is underlying illness, referral should be made to the paediatrician or general practitioner (GP) immediately. A breastfeeding assessment should be taken to identify problems that may have reduced the milk supply or slowed down the onset of lactogenesis II. The most common cause for poor weight gain or weight loss is ineffective removal of milk from the breast, and therefore observation of a breastfeed must be carried out to exclude causes of insufficient milk supply.

Signs of ineffective milk transfer in an infant are:

- Weight loss.
- Abnormal urine or stool output.
- Lethargy and irritability.
- Unsettled infant, particularly after prolonged or frequent feeds.
- Prolonged or excessive jaundice.

Some of the causes of ineffective milk transfer may be:

- Poor position and attachment at the breast.
- Lack of stimulation of the breast – scheduled feeding rather than demand, supplementary feeding, use of teats and dummies.
- Cracked nipples, mastitis or other common problems.

- Maternal issues such as ill health following a traumatic birth or medical problem, caesarean section, retained placenta, polycystic ovaries, obesity, taking the combined contraceptive pill, substance abuse, previous breast surgery.
- Lack of confidence.

Monitoring weight

A healthy infant should be weighed naked at birth and around the fifth and tenth days as part of the assessment of feeding to ensure the birth weight is regained. However, weighing will occur more frequently if the infant is preterm, having feeding problems or has an underlying illness. Iyer *et al.* (2008) found that early weighing with appropriate lactation support resulted in earlier identification of problems, such as neonatal hypernatraemic dehydration, and led to higher breastfeeding rates. Weight loss is calculated as a percentage using the following formula:

$$\frac{\text{weight loss (g)}}{\text{birth weight(g)}} \times 100 = \text{weight loss}(\%)$$

Therefore, if the birth weight is 3800 g, the weight loss will be:

$$\frac{200\text{g}}{3800\text{g}} \times 100 = 5.2(\%)$$

Weight should be plotted on the Royal College of Paediatrics and Child Health (RCPCH) UK-WHO growth charts (2013), which include a separate preterm section for infants 32–36 weeks' gestation and a chart for preterm infants born from 23 weeks' gestation (www.rcpch.ac.uk/resources/uk-who-growth-charts-0-4-years).

To ensure accurate weight recording, the following guidelines should be followed:

- Use class III electronic/digital scales.
- Weigh babies when they are naked.
- Place scales on a hard surface.
- The infant should be naked in a prone position.
- Weigh before a feed.
- When possible, use the same scales.
- Weighing scales should be serviced annually.

Management of weight loss or poor weight gain

Weight loss or poor weight gain of 10 per cent or less

(See local policies as there may be some difference.)

- Take a breastfeeding assessment and observe a breastfeed and sucking pattern.
- Correct specific problems that have led to weight loss or poor weight gain.
- Encourage prolonged skin-to-skin contact and rooming-in.
- Teach skills of position and attachment, feeding pattern and recognising infant feeding cues.

- Stimulate the breast with regular breastfeeding and/or expressing every two to three hours.
- Supplementary feeds may be required. These should be in the form of expressed breast-milk following a breastfeed when possible.
- Avoid teats and dummies.
- Closely monitor urine and stool output and feeding behaviour.
- Reweigh in two to three days.

Practice recommendations: newborn weight management

In newborns, a normal weight loss is considered to be less than 10 per cent, and most infants regain their birth weight within three weeks of birth. Weight loss over 10 per cent of the birth weight is indicative that the infant is not getting enough milk. If by three weeks of age the infant has not regained her or his birth weight, the mother should be referred to an experienced infant feeding adviser and paediatrician (NICE, 2018b). Clear communication and documentation regarding the plan of care between the healthcare professionals is required as this is often the time when the care of the mother and infant is transferred to the health visitor. The aims of the intervention are to increase the mother's confidence and motivation to continue breastfeeding, to address and correct the identified problem and prevent further complications.

Weight loss of 10–12 per cent

- As above.
- Exclude illness or infection.
- Refer to paediatrician or GP as appropriate.
- Encourage the mother to express milk after every feed at the breast and then cup feed. Donor or formula milk may be required if insufficient expressed breastmilk is available.
- Consider switch feeding and additional support from the breastfeeding team.
- Weigh in 24–48 hours.

Weight loss greater than 12 per cent

- As above.
- Refer to the neonatal unit and paediatric staff, to be seen by an experienced infant feeding adviser.

If weight loss is above 15 per cent, an emergency paediatric review is required. A full biochemical profile for electrolytes and renal function will be performed as well as a renal ultrasound. If the infant is able to breastfeed, this should continue; however, intravenous fluids will also be required. The mother should be reviewed by a skilled breastfeeding adviser and encouraged to express breastmilk every two to three hours. Donor milk or formula may be required if insufficient expressed breastmilk.

Activity

Ensure you are familiar with your local policy for weighing infants and the referral process should it be required. What are the differences in the policy for normal healthy term infants and those in the neonatal unit?

Practice recommendations: older infant weight management

In the first four months of life, an infant will gain approximately 125–200 g per week. This will slow down to 50–150 g by four to six months and 25–75 g by six to 12 months. This varies between infants, but similar methods of ensuring the newborn is thriving can be applied to the older child:

- The infant is active and alert.
- At least six wet nappies a day.
- Frequent stools.
- Good signs of position and attachment at the breast.

Poor weight gain can be attributed to underlying illness; however, it is more commonly due to poor breastfeeding technique or problems with lactation. Management will include a full breastfeeding assessment, observation of position and attachment, monitoring of urine and stool output, observation of feeding behaviour, and skilled help and support. Skin-to-skin contact and co-bathing should be advised at any age to encourage feeding behaviour. The mother may also need to increase the number of times she breastfeeds and to express following a feed to increase her milk supply (see Chapter 4).

Faltering growth

After the first two weeks, it is recommended that weighing occurs no more than once a month up to 6 months of age, no more than once a month from 6–12 months of age and no more than once every 3 months over the age of 1. However, if there is concern, the infant should be weighed more frequently, and a clinical, developmental and social assessment should be performed as well as a detailed feeding history and observation of a feed (NICE, 2017).

Weight should be plotted on the RCPCH growth charts. NICE (2017) suggest using the following thresholds for concern about faltering growth in babies

- A fall across one or more weight centile spaces if birth weight was below the 9th centile.
- A fall across two or more weight centile spaces if birth weight was between the 9th and 91st centiles.
- A fall across three or more centile spaces if birth weight was above the 91st centile.
- When current weight is below the second centile for age, whatever the birth weight.

In addition, length or height should be measured if there are concerns about a child's weight gain, growth or general health. Appropriate referral to other professionals should be made as required.

Hypernatraemic dehydration

All infants are expected to lose weight within the first few days of life, which is thought to be due to fluid loss. A normal weight loss is currently considered to be up to 7 per cent of the birth weight. Extreme weight loss is, however, associated with hypernatraemic dehydration – increased blood sodium levels – and is usually caused by insufficient feeding (Dewey *et al.*, 2005; Osman *et al.*, 2021).

All healthcare professionals must be aware of the signs of hypernatraemia:

- Weight loss.
- Abnormal pattern of wet and dirty nappies.
- Lethargy or irritability.
- Fever.
- Jaundice.

It must be noted that newborn infants with hypernatraemic dehydration do not always display the classical signs of dehydration, for example, increased skin turgor, sunken fontanelle, sunken eyes, dry mucous membranes, increased capillary refill time and cool and blue peripheries. These may all be absent, but the infant may still be dehydrated. It is therefore essential to teach mothers what the normal pattern of feeding is and what they can expect. Infants older than 48 hours old usually feed approximately eight times in 24 hours (hypernatraemia is rare in infants younger than 48 hours old). Livingstone *et al.* (2000) gave the risk factors for hypernatraemic dehydration as:

- Abnormalities of the mouth.
- Preterm infants.
- Use of teats or pacifiers.
- Birth trauma.
- Medical problems.
- Separation from mother.
- Sleepy baby.

Mother

- Breast problems such as cracked nipples, hypoplasia.
- Complicated birth.
- Delayed lactogenesis II.
- Postpartum haemorrhage.
- Infrequent breast stimulation.

If infant weight loss is greater than 7 per cent and continues to fall within the first week of life or the birth weight has not been regained by the tenth day, referral should be made to a skilled infant feeding adviser for the early detection of insufficient milk transfer and the prevention of hypernatraemic dehydration. If not treated appropriately, it can have severe consequences such as jaundice, cerebral oedema, convulsions, acute renal failure, brain damage and death (Osman, 2021).

Vitamin D supplementation

There has been great debate in recent years regarding whether or not breastfed infants require vitamin supplementation, in particular vitamin D. Vitamin D is predominantly produced photochemically in the skin by exposure to sunlight and is available in a few foods (e.g. fish oils, liver, dairy products). Due to concerns about vitamin D deficiency, some countries fortify foods such as cereals, bread and margarine.

Vitamin D regulates calcium phosphate, which is essential for the development of healthy bones. It is associated with protection against prostate and colon cancer, psoriasis and a number of autoimmune disorders, as well as a reduction in the incidence of type 1 diabetes. Deficiency is associated with increased susceptibility to tuberculosis, cardiovascular disease, some cancers and osteomalacia. In infants, a deficiency results in rickets and continues to be a problem in some high-risk groups (SACN, 2016). People with darker skin pigmentation, such as Black and Asian ethnic minority groups, and those with lifestyle and cultural practices that reduce the amount of time their skin is exposed to sunlight are at greater risk of vitamin D deficiency (Ladhani *et al.*, 2004).

In response to a request by the Department of Health, SACN (2016, 2018) published the following new recommendation on vitamin D. The aim is to ensure the majority of the UK population has satisfactory vitamin D levels all year round.

- All babies from birth up to one year of age should consume 8.5 micrograms of vitamin D per day and 10 micrograms for ages one to four years.
- Everyone in the general population over four years of age should consume 10 micrograms of vitamin D daily. This includes pregnant and lactating women and at-risk population groups.

All women should be informed at the booking appointment about the importance of their own and their infant's health of maintaining adequate vitamin D stores during pregnancy and whilst breastfeeding. As breastmilk contains low levels of vitamin D, it is important to ensure that breastfed infants are not susceptible to vitamin D deficiency. SACN (2016) were unable to quantify the amount of safe exposure to sunlight that is required to synthesise vitamin D, but the previous recommendation was approximately 15 minutes three times a week from April to September for people with fair skin and slightly more for those with darker pigmentation (avoiding excessive exposure to sunlight to minimise the risk of skin cancer) for mother and infant. In colder climates during winter, there is not enough sunlight to maintain vitamin D.

Discharge planning

Support with breastfeeding must continue following discharge from the neonatal unit. An individualised care plan should be developed prior to discharge and communicated to the healthcare team that will be providing future care and support; this may be the midwife or health visitor. Any equipment such as breast pumps, storage bottles and sterilising equipment should be in situ before the infant goes home, and the mother should have been shown how to work and maintain the pump as well as safely express and store breastmilk. Follow-up appointments should be made to assess feeding and to ensure the infant is thriving. The mother should also be informed about other mechanisms of support, such as help lines, support groups, peer supporters and specialist infant feeding advisers (see Chapter 11).

Concluding comments

There are many situations when breastfeeding can be challenging, but this is particularly the case when an infant has special needs or requirements. It is clear from the evidence that breastmilk offers protection from further illness, and healthcare professionals must offer a coordinated approach to care both in the hospital environment and on discharge home.

Scenarios

What would you recommend in the following situations?

1 Amy is three days old and has been prescribed phototherapy for jaundice. Her mother, Carol, informs you that Amy is not feeding well, and a friend has advised her to give formula milk as well as breastfeed to clear the jaundice.
2 Lizzie has come to you today. Her baby, Frank, is 10 weeks old. Frank was 3.5 kg born at 40 weeks' gestation, on the 50th centile. Now Frank's weight is 4.5 kg, which is on the ninth centile. Lizzie says feeding is erratic, and Frank has to be 'topped up' with formula milk, as the feeds are sometimes 'frantic', and he keeps coming off the breast.

Further reading

- Inherited Metabolic Disorders in Scotland (IMD Scotland) www.imd.scot.nhs. uk BLISS for babies born premature or sick www.bliss.org.uk.
- RCPCH UK-WHO growth charts- 0–4 years www.rcpch.ac.uk/resources/uk-who-growth-charts-0-4-years.
- Pregnant women and mothers with children younger than the age of four years who are on benefits can get Healthy Start vouchers to spend on milk, fruit and vegetables as well as vitamins. Further details are available at www.healthystart. nhs.uk.
- SACN (Scientific Advisory Committee on Nutrition) (2016) Vitamin D and Health is available online at www.gov.uk/government/groups/scientific-advisory-committee-on-nutrition.

9 Alternative methods of infant feeding when breastfeeding is not possible

- Learning outcomes
- Supplementary and complementary feeding
- Alternatives to breastfeeding
- Donor milk
- Formula feeding
- Sterilisation, preparation and reconstitution of formula milk
- Concluding comments
- Reflective questions
- Resources

It is important to acknowledge that, in some circumstances, breastfeeding is not possible for mothers or infants. This chapter covers a range of alternative feeding methods and the use of donor milk when the mother's own breastmilk is not available. Safe artificial feeding is also described and instruction on sterilising feeding equipment included.

Learning outcomes

By the end of this chapter, you will be able to:

- identify alternative methods of infant feeding when feeding at the breast is not possible, including the use of expressed breastmilk, donor breastmilk and formula milk;
- discuss the risks and benefits of alternative methods of feeding;
- demonstrate how to feed an infant safely with these alternative methods; and
- demonstrate how to prepare formula milk safely and sterilise feeding equipment.

Mapping to UNICEF Baby Friendly Initiative (BFI) Education learning outcomes (2019a)
    By the end of the programme, students will:

Theme		Learning outcomes
Theme 2: Support infant feeding	6.	Have the knowledge and skills to support mothers and babies to maximise breastmilk and breastfeeding, to continue to breastfeed for as long as they wish and to introduce solid foods at an appropriate time.

DOI: 10.4324/9781003282341-9

Theme		Learning outcomes
	7.	Be able to support parents who formula feed to do so responsively and as safely as possible.
Theme 4: Manage the challenges	12.	Have an understanding of the special circumstances which can affect lactation and breastfeeding (e.g. when mother and baby are separated, including preterm and sick infants) and be able to support mothers to overcome the challenges.
Theme 5: Promote positive communication	14.	Have an understanding of the principles of effective communication and current thinking around public health promotion strategies and approaches.

The best way for infants to receive breastmilk is to suckle at the breast. However, sometimes breastfeeding is not possible due to a variety of reasons such as illness, prematurity or separation from the mother. It is therefore essential that healthcare professionals not only have a sound knowledge of the available alternative methods of feeding but also know how to assess the appropriateness for the gestational age and clinical condition of the infant.

Nipple confusion is a major concern for healthcare professionals as well as a point of controversy and can be defined as the interference of artificial nipples, such as teats and dummies or pacifiers, with the successful initiation of breastfeeding. It is this idea that formed the basis of the original Step 9 of the UNICEF *Ten Steps* (WHO, 1998a): 'Give no artificial teats or dummies to breastfeeding infants', updated in 2017 to 'Counsel mothers on the use and risks of feeding bottles, teats and pacifiers'. It is clear that there is a difference in the mechanism of sucking an artificial teat and the breast; however, there is limited evidence to support the avoidance of teats or dummies in healthy term infants, and much of the research available is based on premature infants or infants with other compounding factors rather than healthy term infants (Zimmerman and Thompson, 2015; Jaafar *et al.*, 2016a).

As there is no way of determining which infants will develop nipple confusion, it is appropriate to avoid artificial teats where possible and use other devices until the infant is able to feed from the breast, for example by nasogastric tube, cup, spoon or supplementer (see Table 9.1 for examples that may be used at different gestational ages).

Supplementary and complementary feeding

'Supplementary feeding' and 'complementary feeding' are terms that are often used interchangeably, but they mean very different things. In some literature, 'supplementary'

Table 9.1 Suggested feeding devices suitable for gestational age and feeding behaviour

Gestational age (weeks)	Feeding behaviour	Suggested feeding device for supplement
<30–32	Uncoordinated suck-swallow-breathe reflex	Intravenous gastric tube
30–32	Can 'lap' milk	Drops of milk; cup feed
32	Begins to suckle at the breast but requires supplementation	Cup feed; supplementer
34–36	Increasing amounts from breast	Cup feed

means giving a feed in place of a breastfeed, whereas 'complementary' means topping up a breastfeed with expressed breastmilk, formula or even water. The following UNICEF UK BFI definitions are used in this book:

- *Supplementary feeding*: Feeds given to an infant younger than six months old to supplement the intake of breastmilk, when this is insufficient.
- *Complementary feeding*: The introduction of foods and drinks after six months of age. These foods are in addition to an adequate intake of breastmilk.

The *Infant Feeding Survey 2010* (McAndrew *et al.*, 2012) reported that 92 per cent of mothers had decided how they were going to feed their infants before birth; 75 per cent planned to breastfeed, an increase of 5 per cent from the 2005 *Infant Feeding Survey* (Bolling *et al.*, 2007); 14 per cent of whom had decided to both breastfeed and bottle feed. The 2017 *Scottish Maternal and Infant Nutrition Survey* similarly found 94 per cent of mothers had decided how they would feed their infants before birth. However, of the 74 per cent who said they intended to give breastmilk, 42 per cent intended to exclusively breastfeed, 18 per cent to combine breast and expressing and 14 per cent to combine breast and formula milk. Twenty per cent intended to formula feed. Overall, those who had declared how they would feed their babies did so, and of the 6 per cent who were undecided, 64 per cent gave breastmilk at some point, as did 5 per cent of those who decided to formula feed.

Those who had ever given breastmilk were asked whether they had ever given their babies any infant formula. Overall, two-thirds of these respondents (66 per cent) had given some formula milk to their babies, 33 per cent within the first 48 hours, 17 per cent within two weeks and 16 per cent more than two weeks after the birth. The most common reasons can be found in Table 9.2. Other reasons offered included were the baby being premature or in special care (5 per cent), the mother or baby being unwell (3 per cent) or the baby having hypoglycaemia (3 per cent).

If supplementation is considered necessary, it must be preceded by making a breastfeeding assessment and observing a breastfeed. Breastmilk should always be used as the preferred option to formula milk where available.

Table 9.2 Reasons for giving formula milk

Reason	In hospital or within 48 hours (%)	Within 2 weeks (%)	After 2 weeks (%)
I had problems breastfeeding	49	61	28
A health professional advised me	36	34	11
Anxious about how much milk baby getting	31	44	23
I always intended to mix feed	21	17	17
Previous experience with another baby	14	15	14
It allowed my partner to be involved	13	22	31
To make breastfeeding more manageable	12	18	33
To help my baby to sleep longer	7	10	16
Partner/friend/relative advised me	6	10	10
Attending social event	2	3	16
Other reason	18	5	19

Source: Scottish Maternal and Infant Nutrition Survey 2017, Q42, 8–12 Week Survey

It is helpful to inform parents what the capacity of a newborn's stomach is as because a common cause of anxiety is that they are not getting enough milk and therefore may overfeed (Figure 9.1).

To guide healthcare professionals, the WHO and UNICEF (2009) published the following guidelines for acceptable medical reasons for giving breastmilk substitutes:

- **Infants with the following conditions cannot have breastmilk and require specialised formula milk:**

  - Galactasaemia (need galactose-free formula).
  - Maple syrup urine disease (need formula free of leucine, isoleucine and valine).
  - Phenylketonuria (breastfeeding is possible but they also need phenylalanine-free formula and close expert monitoring) (See Chapter 8 for further details.)

- **Infants may need other food in addition to breastmilk for a limited period if they are:**

  - Born weighing less than 1,500 g.
  - Born at less than 32 weeks' gestational age.
  - At risk of hypoglycaemia (preterm, small for gestational age, have had a hypoxic episode, are ill infants or infants whose mothers are diabetic, with low blood sugar levels) (See Chapter 8 for further details.)

If the mother is positive for human immunodeficiency syndrome, breastfeeding should be avoided if suitable alternatives are available (see Chapter 7). Some other conditions require breastfeeding to cease temporarily, but it can resume if or when there is a change in status, for example, severe illness such as sepsis; herpes simplex lesions on the breast; taking medications such as sedatives, anti-epileptic drugs and other drugs that could cause drowsiness; and radioactive iodine or chemotherapy (see Chapter 7).

Other issues that could indicate supplementation are geographic separation, delayed lactogenesis II, severe nipple pain, breast anomalies or previous breast surgery, infant

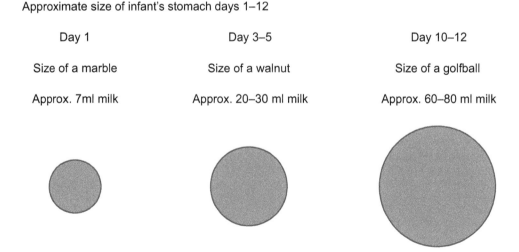

Approximate size of infant's stomach days 1–12

Day 1	Day 3–5	Day 10–12
Size of a marble	Size of a walnut	Size of a golfball
Approx. 7ml milk	Approx. 20–30 ml milk	Approx. 60–80 ml milk

Figure 9.1 Newborn stomach size

dehydration, weight loss of more than 7–10 per cent of the birth weight and meconium still present at five days (see Chapters 6, 7, 8 for mor information).

To ensure lactation is maintained and improved in these situations, mothers should be encouraged to have skin-to-skin contact, attempt to breastfeed when possible and express breastmilk after the attempted breastfeed to encourage prolactin production and avoid a build-up of the feedback inhibitor of lactation (see Chapter 3), which will reduce the milk supply and trigger apoptosis.

Alternatives to breastfeeding

Nasogastric tube feeding

Nasogastric tube feeding is used to provide breast or formula milk for premature or ill infants when the infant cannot maintain its nutritional needs via the breast or bottle alone or due to a lack of ability to suckle adequately. The nasogastric tube delivers the milk straight into the stomach, and therefore the infant does not have the oral stimulus of the feed. It is preferable if a bolus feed is administered during kangaroo care or when the infant is at the breast, even if the infant cannot suck, so that they associate the feed with the breast.

Procedure for inserting the tube and delivering the milk

- Measure the tube from the tip of the xiphisternum to the tragus of the ear (tough fold of cartilage at the entrance to the ear) and to the nostrils.
- The infant should be relaxed.
- Insert the tube slowly to avoid vagal stimulation and resulting bradycardia.
- Check for gastric aspirate using pH indicator paper to ensure the tube is in the stomach not the lungs. Gastric contents should be pH 5.5 or less. A pH above 6 could indicate the tube is in the intestines; a pH above 7 could indicate the tube is in the lungs and must be removed.

Once it has been confirmed that the tube is in the correct position, feeding can commence. An oral syringe should be used to administer the feed. The milk should be delivered using gravity, not pushed down the tube with a plunger. Always refer to local guidelines.

Cup feeding

From approximately 30 weeks' gestation, infants have the ability to lap milk from a cup. The advantages of cup feeding for preterm infants above other methods such as a nasogastric tube are that it provides oral and gastric stimulation. The infant experiences taste and demonstrates tongue movement. With cup feeding, the infant is able to control the amount and rate of the feed similarly to breastfeeding; therefore, the intake for preterm infants should be monitored over a 24-hour period rather than forcing the calculated amount at each feed. It is also important to note that, compared with bottle feeding, preterm infants who are cup fed have higher oxygen saturation levels and are less likely to desaturate during a feed, and they also have lower heart rates (Penny *et al.*, 2018). However, cup feeding is not appropriate for all infants; it is unsuitable for infants who have a poor gag reflex or are lethargic, as they are likely to aspirate.

Flint *et al.* (2016) conducted a review of five studies that compared cup and bottle feeding in preterm infants. They concluded that infants fed by cup were more likely to be exclusively breastfeeding at discharge, three months and six months than those who were bottle fed. However, there is a dearth of evidence about cup feeding, as established by McKinney *et al.* (2016), who conducted a review of the literature. Whilst there appeared to be a higher proportion of cup-fed infants reported to have any breastfeeding and exclusive breastfeeding on discharge than those given a bottle, they continued to identify the need for further research.

Procedure for cup feeding

- Wrap the infant and support the infant in an upright position.
- Half fill the cup with breastmilk or formula.
- Bring the brim of the cup to the outer corners of the infant's upper lip, resting on the lower lip.
- Tip the cup to ensure the milk is touching the infant's lips so the infant can lap or sip the milk. Do not pour the milk into the mouth.
- Allow the infant to regulate the pace but avoid the feeding session taking over 30 minutes.
- Keep the cup in position while the infant rests.
- Wind the infant at regular intervals.

Always refer to local guidelines.

Syringe

Small doses of approximately 0.5 ml via a 1-ml syringe may be suitable for infants who can swallow but not suck; any amounts greater than this should be administered via a cup to avoid aspiration.

Procedure for syringe feeding

- Wrap the infant and support the infant in an upright position.
- Deliver very small amounts of milk into the cheek area of the mouth.
- Allow time for the infant to swallow and take a breath in between each dose.

Always refer to local guidelines.

Breastfeeding supplementer

The supplementer is a fine tube that, when attached to the breast, is used to supplement feeding during a breastfeed (Figure 9.2). As the infant takes the breast into her or his mouth, she or he also takes the tube. As the flow of milk at the breast is stronger than the tube, the infant first empties the breast and then receives the prescribed supplement. The benefits of this device are that it enables the infant to suckle at the breast and obtain breastmilk on demand, providing a positive feeding experience for mother and infant while stimulating lactogenesis. It encourages a baby who is reluctant to suckle, has sucking problems or is unwell. In addition, the supplementer can be used to breastfeed as a non-birth parent.

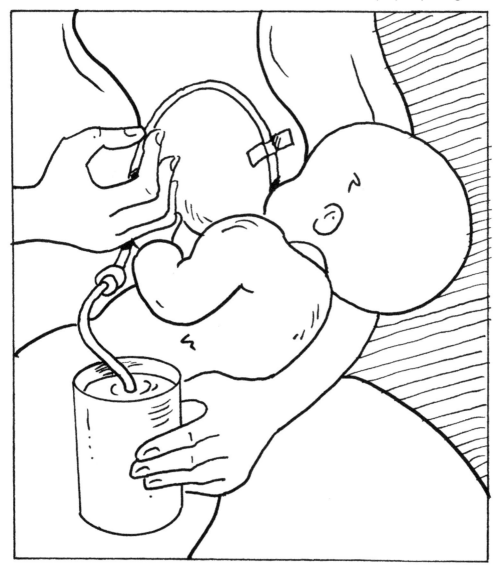

Figure 9.2 A breastfeeding supplementer

The supplementer facilitates delivery of nutrition for the infant while stimulating the breast to produce milk and is therefore suitable for mothers with insufficient milk supply, those who have had prior breast surgery, to help induce lactation or relactation, and for mothers with premature infants or infants with disorders, illness or neurological impairment that cause a weak suck.

Procedure for using a breastfeeding supplementer

- Use a fine tube such as a nasogastric tube and a cup or bag for the milk (expressed breastmilk when possible).

- Place one end of the tube along the nipple so that the infant suckles the breast and tube at the same time.
- Place the other end of the tube in the cup of milk or attach it to the bag.
- Control the milk flow by raising the cup to increase the flow and lowering it to decrease the flow.
- Thoroughly clean the equipment between each use by boiling or sterilising or, if in hospital, use single-use equipment.

Finger feeding

Finger feeding is when a feeding tube is attached to the finger and inserted in the infant's mouth. It is a useful method for mothers who experience breast refusal or whose infant is sleepy, has latching problems or is premature with suckling difficulties. It is most commonly used to prepare and encourage the infant to feed at the breast.

Procedure for finger feeding

- Use a suitable container to hold the milk and attach the tube securely.
- Place the tube so that it is placed on the soft part of the index (or other) finger.
- The end of the tube should go no further than the end of the finger. Taping it to the finger may help it maintain position.
- Wrap the infant and support the infant in an upright position.
- Using the finger with the tube attached, gently touch the infant's lips until the mouth opens. The infant should begin to suckle.
- The soft part of the finger should be flat and face upwards towards the roof of the mouth.
- If feeding is very slow, the container may be raised above the infant's head.

Haberman feeder

A Haberman feeder is a special bottle developed for infants with impaired sucking ability (e.g. cleft lip and palate). It is designed to mimic breastfeeding as opposed to sucking on a traditional artificial teat and bottle.

Dropper or pipette

These devices may be used to drop milk on to the breast to encourage the infant to suckle or lick at the breast. This is useful for reluctant feeders and premature infants who are unable to suck and to encourage the let-down reflex.

Donor milk

Donor milk banking was established to collect, screen, pasteurise and distribute donated breastmilk for infants whose mothers are unable to breastfeed or supply their own breastmilk. In 2010, NICE developed donor breastmilk guidelines aimed at professionals who support mothers who use donor milk, work in a donor milk bank or intend to set up a donor milk bank. At the time of publishing, there were only 14 donor breastmilk banks in the UK that supplied breastmilk predominantly for infants requiring neonatal care.

The United Kingdom Association for Milk Banking (UKAMB) is a registered charity that supports donor milk banking and is a useful resource for parents and professionals (see www.ukamb.org).

Potential donors go through a rigorous screening interview and serological testing at enrolment. Donors are given information on the processes and how the breastmilk will be used and are informed that it will not be returned to them. Informed consent is gained before any breastmilk is provided.

During the screening interview, the donor is asked if she smokes; drinks more than two units of alcohol twice a week; uses or has ever used recreational drugs; has ever tested positive for HIV, hepatitis B or C, human T-lymphotrophic virus or syphilis; or is at increased risk of Creutzfeldt-Jacob disease. If she answers 'yes' to any of these questions, she is not allowed to donate her breastmilk. If she answers 'no' to the questions, she undergoes serological screening and another interview. Donors require ongoing training, support and assessment of health and serological status. They are advised to contact the milk bank if they develop pyrexia, take medication or develop any breast infection, including mastitis.

NICE *Donor milk banks, CG 93* (2010 (reviewed 2018)) provides further information. Training for donors includes:

- The importance of hand washing and good technique.
- Personal hygiene.
- Expressing and collecting breastmilk.
- Cleaning and using breast pumps.
- storing breastmilk (including labelling and documentation).
- Transporting the breastmilk.

Donors are encouraged to express milk by hand and collect the expressed milk rather than 'drip' milk (milk that drips from one breast while the infant is feeding at the other). The NICE guideline (NICE, 2010) provides strict criteria for the storage, collection, transport and processing of donor milk. The donor milk is pasteurised at 62.5°C for 30 minutes and can be stored for no longer than six months. Good documentation of all the processes is kept for 30 years after the expiry date. Donor breastmilk is only supplied to hospitals that agree to comply with the tracking process.

Donor milk usually comes from mothers who have given birth at term. Therefore, the milk content tends to be variable in relation to fat, energy and protein content and alone may not meet the nutritional requirements of preterm or low birth weight infants. However, donor breastmilk does have the advantage of providing the immunoprotective factors and growth factors that may prevent necrotising enterocolitis (NEC). Quigley *et al.* (2019) conducted a systematic review and found that although there were greater short-term growth rates in preterm infants fed with formula, it was associated with an increased incidence of NEC.

Administering donor milk in the neonatal unit

All donor breastmilk (or mothers' own expressed milk) should be checked by two members of staff beside the infant immediately prior to administration. The infant's name and identifying number should be checked against the milk and the infant. The staff should also ensure that consent has been gained from the parents. The consent form, alongside the donor milk record sheet, should be kept with the infant's case record and a copy sent to the donor milk bank for tracking purposes.

Activity

Does your local neonatal unit use donor breastmilk? Read the local policy and guidelines as there may be slight variation in procedure.

Formula feeding

Although breastmilk is the gold standard for infant nutrition, some mothers are unable to, or choose not to, breastfeed or express breastmilk for their infants. The only alternative to breastmilk suitable for infants younger than one year is formula milk (NHS, 2018). It is therefore essential that healthcare professionals support these mothers and have knowledge about formula milks. In the past, the message from UNICEF UK BFI was sometimes misconstrued, and some healthcare professionals falsely believed that the BFI did not allow them to advise and support women who choose to bottle feed. This was never the case; however, they addressed this concern in recent standards (UNICEF UK BFI, 2017a) in which it is clear that the aim of the BFI is to support the development of strong relationships between mother and infant to give infants the best start in life.

Formula milks are designed to be similar to breastmilk. However, because of the nature of breastmilk (see Chapter 3), formula milk cannot replicate it fully (Table 9.3). Most formula milks are developed from cow's milk; however, soya milk is also available to parents.

UK regulations governing the composition and marketing of formula milks changed in 2020 when the EU directive Foods for Specific Groups (609/2013) came into force. Formula and infant milks must be marketed as foods for special medical purposes. Further detailed information can be found at Commission Delegated Regulation (EU) 2016/127 (supplementing Regulation (EU) No 609/2013): guidance – GOV.UK (www.gov.uk). The regulations regarding the marketing and labelling of formula milks applies across the UK. There may be some variations in the permitted content between formula brands, and

Table 9.3 Comparison of breast and formula milk

Nutrient	Breastmilk	Formula milk
Fat	Omega docosahexaenoic acid (DHA), arachidonic acid	No DHA
	Cholesterol	No cholesterol
	Lipase	No lipase
	Adjusts to infant's needs, reducing as infant gets older	Does not adjust
Protein	Increase in whey (easy to digest)	Increase in curds (harder to digest)
	Lactoferrin (binds iron)	No lactoferrin
	Lysosomes	No lysosomes
	Immunoglobulin A (IgA)	No IgA
Carbohydrate	Lactose (important for brain development)	Deficient in lactose
	Rich in oligosaccharides	Deficient in oligosaccharides
Other	Taste varies	Taste never varies

Source: Adapted from RCM (2009)

these can cause intolerance in some infants. If this is the case, mothers can change the brand, usually under the advice of the midwife or health visitor. There are no regulations related to composition, marketing or labelling of milks for those marketed for children older than 12 months.

Types of formula milk

Preterm milk

These products are designed to provide nutrients suitable for preterm infants and are enriched with proteins and minerals.

First milks

These are for newborns and are based on the whey of cow's milk at a ratio of 60:40 whey:casein, which is similar to breastmilk. Whey-dominant formula is more easily digested than casein-dominant formulas. First milks are suitable for most infants until they are one year old, when full-fat cow's milk can be introduced (NHS, 2019a).

Hungrier baby formula

The main difference from first milks is that 'hungrier baby milks' are casein dominant, the ratio being 20:80 whey:casein. They are marketed for 'hungry infants', and manufacturers state that they *can* be given to newborns, but the high casein ratio, which is supposed to make the infant feel full and settle more easily, makes them more difficult to digest, and they are therefore not usually recommended for newborns by healthcare professionals. NHS (2019a) recommends continuing whey-based formula milk or first milk until the age of 12 months.

Follow-on milks

These milks are marketed as suitable for infants older than six months of age and should never be used in younger infants. They contain more iron, sugars and minerals than first milks. There is no evidence to suggest any benefits for infants moving to follow-on formula at six months, and therefore it is not recommended (NHS, 2019a; PHS, 2021).

Goodnight milks

These milks are marketed for infants between the ages of six months and three years and contain follow-on milk with rice flour, whole-grain oatmeal and corn starch. They can be given via a bottle or feeding cup. Again, on behalf of the Department of Health, SACN (2008, p. 3) could find no evidence to support manufacturers' claims that they 'settle the infant for the night' or are 'gentler on the infant's tummy'. SACN (2008, pp. 3–4) identified some other concerns about these milks:

- They may replace the night breastfeed, therefore undermining continued breastfeeding.
- Going to bed immediately after such a feed could result in prolonged tooth exposure to the food and lead to dental caries. (The manufacturers do recommend brushing the teeth before bed; however, this seems to contradict the notion of 'settling' the infant.)

- Some parents may use these formula feeds to settle the infant at other times of the day, and this may interfere with weaning. SACN suggests that they are not a suitable alternative to meals.
- The preparation of goodnight milks is different from those of other formula milks and may cause confusion for parents.

NHS (2019a) states there is no evidence suggest this type of formula is needed.

Soya milk

This is made from soya beans and is not advised as an alternative milk for infants; it should only be used under the advice of a general practitioner or health visitor. Despite common perception, infants who are allergic to cow's milk may also be allergic to soya milk, and it cannot be recommended for the prevention of allergies (FSA, 2013). Soya milk contains high levels of phytoestrogen, which may pose long-term reproductive problems. It may also cause problems for infants with hypothyroidism and stimulate allergies. Soya milk contains more sugars from non-milk sources and can therefore lead to dental caries. Martyn (2003) suggested that infants of parents who are vegans are most at risk, as they may assume that the infant will get the same benefits as adults. In conclusion, the FSA (2013, p. 24) stated and reasserted in 2021 (FSA, 2021), 'There is no scientific basis for a change in the current government advice that there is no substantive medical need for, nor health benefit arising from the use of soya-based infant formula and it should only be used in exceptional circumstances to ensure adequate nutrition'.

Other formula milks

Goat's milk formula is not suitable for infants. Hypoallergenic formulas for infants with a proven cow's milk intolerance or at risk of allergies should be used under medical or dietetic consultation.

Full-fat cow's milk

This should not be given to infants younger than one year of age.

Key facts

Although goat's and cow's milk should not be given as a drink before the age of one year, small amounts of pasteurised cow's milk can be used in preparing foods for infants older than six months.

Full-fat dairy products such as yogurt can be given after six months (NHS, 2019a).

Constituents of formula milk

- *Long-chain fatty acids* are found in breastmilk and are thought to improve brain and eye development. Formula manufacturers introduced them into their milk and use them to market their products. However, Simmer *et al.* (2017) found no evidence of benefit or harm when added to formula.

- Infant formula companies have introduced *prebiotics* into their milk in an attempt to encourage the growth of 'good bacteria', bifidobacteria and lactobacilli, in the digestive tract or the good bacteria in the form of *probiotics*. Osborn and Sinn (2013) conducted a systematic review and found some evidence that prebiotic supplement in formula milk could prevent eczema but caution that further research is needed.
- *Nucleotides* make up the units of DNA and RNA and are thought to enhance gastro-intestinal and immunological effects.
- *Vitamins A and D* are added to formula milk, including special preterm products, and therefore exclusively formula-fed infants younger than six months of age do not require these supplements. Those older than the age of six months and up to the age of two years require vitamin A, D and C supplements. However, groups at high risk of vitamin D deficiency should still take the supplements (see Chapter 8).
- Formula milk has five to six times more *iron* than breastmilk, but because it is 'free iron' it is less bio-available or readily absorbed and increases the risk of infection.

Advice for parents

The preparation and reconstitution of formula milk, as well as the timings and quantities, can be of great concern to parents, especially if their infants do not adhere to the guidelines on the packet. In the first few days, infants may only take a small amount of formula, but by the end of the first week, they will require approximately 150–200 ml/kg/day until they are six months old. Parents need advice that they should not overfeed their infants in the hope that they will go longer between feeds because infants are likely to vomit and also put on too much weight. Teaching parents the signs to look for when their infants are hungry is helpful.

Signs of hunger

- Moving the head from side to side, with the tongue protruding.
- Sucking fingers.

Parents should not wait until the infant cries because she or he will become frustrated and not feed as well. It is also important to reinforce to the parents that formula-fed infants' sleep patterns may change, particularly during growth spurts, but that this does not mean that the milk needs to be changed or that weaning should commence; the infant may just require a greater number of feeds for a few days.

Many parents worry about the amount of milk the infant drinks and particularly if he or she is getting enough. They should be taught the signs of adequate feeding to look for (see Chapter 4):

- At least six wet (soaked) nappies a day; clear or pale urine.
- Sticky meconium for the first few days of life followed by pale yellow/yellow-brown stools at least once a day.

The infant's weight should be plotted on the growth chart at regular intervals and discussed with the parents (NICE, 2017).

Many parents who formula feed are concerned about constipation and resort to old wives' tales for remedies. Renfrew *et al.* (2003) reported that reconstitution errors are the most common cause of constipation by putting too much powder in the bottle compared with the volume of water. If this is not the cause, changing the brand of milk may be a solution, as the hardness of the stools is related to unsaturated fatty acids in the stools. This should be discussed with the health visitor. There is no evidence to support giving additional water to improve constipation.

Equipment

Many bottles and teats are designed to replicate the breast; however, this is impossible given the unique nature of the anatomy of individuals' breasts. However, parents do seek advice on these products. Milk should drop out of the teat of an upturned bottle at one drop per second. If the flow is too fast, it will spill out of the infant's mouth, and if too slow, the infant may become frustrated.

Sterilisation, preparation and reconstitution of formula milk

Powdered formula milk is not sterile (ready-to-use cartons are) and can become contaminated by pathogens such as *Enterobacter sakazakii* and *Salmonella* spp. In the past 40 years, there have been between 50 and 60 known cases of infection from powdered formula milk; preterm and low birth weight infants are most at risk (FSA, 2018). The Food Standards Agency (FSA) recommends that healthcare professionals should re-emphasise the importance of good hygiene practices in the preparation and storage of feeds to reduce the risk of illness.

Sterilising feeding equipment

- Wash hands with soap and water.
- Wash feeding equipment in hot soapy water.
- Bottle and teat brushes should be used to clean inside teats and bottles to remove all traces of the formula milk.
- Rinse equipment under a running cold tap.
- Sterilise equipment using preferred method and following the manufacturer's guidelines.
- Leave the bottle until time to make up a feed or fully assemble the bottle with the teat inside and lid on to prevent contamination.
- Wash hands and clean preparation surface where formula milk will be reconstituted.

There are different ways to sterilise infant feeding equipment (NHS, 2019a):

Cold water

- Follow the manufacturer's instructions.
- Leave feeding equipment in the sterilising solution for a minimum of 30 minutes.
- Change the sterilising solution every 24 hours.
- Avoid trapped air in bottles or teats.
- Ensure equipment is fully covered with sterilising solution by using a floating cover.

Steam or microwave

- Follow the manufacturer's instructions including how long you can leave equipment before re-sterilising.
- Openings of bottles and teats should face down in the steriliser.

Boiling

- Ensure safety precautions are taken to avoid scalding and never leave unattended.
- Ensure equipment is suitable for boiling.
- Boil equipment for at least 10 minutes.
- Ensure all items are under the water.

It is essential that hands are washed and the surface where the equipment is reassembled is clean. If bottles are not used immediately, it is best to store them fully assembled with teat and lid in place to avoid re-contamination.

McAndrew *et al.* (2012) reported that steam sterilisers were most popular (67 per cent) followed by microwave (16 per cent) and cold water sterilising solution (9 per cent). This remained similar in the *Scottish Maternal and Infant Nutrition Survey* (SG, 2017) with 59 per cent preferring a steam steriliser, 28 per cent microwave, 13 per cent cold water sterilising solution and 8 per cent boiling the equipment.

Renfrew *et al.* (2008) conducted a systematic review to assess the clinical effectiveness and cost-effectiveness of different methods of cleaning and sterilising infant feeding equipment at home. They concluded that there was a lack of evidence to suggest which method is most effective. However, they did emphasise the importance of hand washing before handling the equipment.

Key Fact

Dishwashers clean feeding equipment, but the temperature is not high enough to sterilise.

Preparation of a formula feed

It is recommended that only one bottle of formula should be made up immediately before a feed, as storage of reconstituted powdered milk may enhance the likelihood of becoming contaminated by pathogens such as *E. sakazakii*, thus increasing the risk of illness (NHS, 2019a);

- Clean the preparation area and wash hands with soap and water.
- Boil fresh tap water in a kettle and allow it to cool to no less than 70°C (less than 30 minutes) because at this temperature, it will kill most bacteria. *Don't use previously boiled, artificially softened or bottled water.*
- Pour the required amount of water into the sterilised bottle.
- Add the exact amount of formula to the water following the manufacturers' guidelines. The wrong amount could cause electrolyte imbalance; too much may cause constipation and dehydration, and too little could cause malnutrition.
- Reassemble the bottle and shake well to ensure the powder has reconstituted.
- Quickly cool under a running cold tap or in a container of cold water.
- The temperature should be lukewarm; test a few drops on the inside of the wrist.
- Discard any formula that has not been used after a feed.

Bottled or 'natural mineral water' should not be used to make up a feed as it may contain high levels of sodium or sulphate. If there is no alternative, the sodium (Na) should be less than 200 milligrams (mg) per litre and sulphate (SO4) no higher than 250 milligrams (mg) per litre. It will also need to be boiled as discussed earlier.

If parents are unable to follow best practice for any reason (e.g. leaving the house, taking bottles to nursery), it is important that they are given advice to prepare and store feeds as safely as possible. Reducing the storage time when possible is recommended, and the following options are advised (FSA, 2013; NHS, 2019a):

- Use prepacked cartons of liquid formula (sterile).
- Alternatively, put the boiled water into a vacuum flask and use it to make up the feed fresh at the time it is required. It is important that the water is warm.
- Take the measured amount of formula in a clean, dry container.
- Take an empty sterilised bottle with cap and retaining ring to be removed when ready to make up the feed.

If this is not possible, parents should be advised as follows:

- If more than one feed is required, always prepare them in separate bottles as stated earlier, not in one container.
- If the prepared feed is not used but left at room temperature, it must be discarded.
- Store the bottles in the back of a fridge, not the door, at a temperature below 5°C. (*E. sakazakii* and *Salmonella* spp. can grow in reconstituted formula if stored above this temperature.)
- The fridge temperature needs close monitoring if the fridge is opened frequently.
- The less time the feed is stored in the fridge, the less risk of contamination by pathogens; this time should never exceed 24 hours in the fridge.

When reheating the bottle if stored in the fridge:

- Only remove from the fridge when required.
- Place in a container of warm water for no longer than 15 minutes; never reheat in a microwave as this causes hot spots.
- Shake the bottle to ensure it has reheated evenly and test a few drops on the inside of the wrist to make sure it is lukewarm.

If the parents need to transport a prepared bottle feed, it should have been cooled in the fridge for at least one hour at less than 5°C and immediately placed in a cool bag with icepacks. It must be used within four hours. If transported in less than four hours, it should be placed in a fridge at less than 5°C and used within 24 hours. If there is no access to a fridge or icepack, the feed must be used within two hours. However, this situation should be avoided when possible and is only advised in exceptional circumstances, as it increases the risk of contamination by pathogens and resulting ill health (NHS, 2019a).

The *Infant Feeding Survey 2010* (McAndrews *et al.*, 2012) reported that almost half of mothers who had prepared formula feeds in the previous seven days had followed the recommendations: (1) making no more than one feed at a time, (2) making feeds within 30 minutes of boiling the water and (3) adding water to the bottle before the powder. This was an increase of 13 per cent compared with 2005. Approximately 65 per cent of mothers said they had followed the recommendations for feeding their infants away from home. This had improved again in the *Scottish Maternal and Infant Nutrition Survey* (SG, 2017) with 71 per cent of respondents reporting they only made one feed at a time.

Responsive bottle feeding

UNICEF UK BFI (2016b, 2019b) promotes responsive bottle feeding but suggests that true responsive feeding is not possible when bottle feeding but is a helpful way for mothers to recognise feeding cues and recommends sensitively explaining that only the parents feed the infant in the early weeks to help the infant to feel safe and secure and to build a close and loving bond.

- Offer feeds when the infant shows signs of hunger.
- If the infant is crying, try to sooth the infant before the feed; skin contact will help.
- Hold the infant close and look into the infant's eyes and talk gently to them.
- Keep the infant in a semi-upright position with their head supported.
- Brush the teat over the lips to encourage an open mouth tongue is poking out.
- Position the bottle horizontally and tilt it so that the infant can get the milk but avoid letting it flowing too fast from the teat.
- Bubbles will be seen in the bottle if the infant is feeding well.
- Observe the infant's cues and allow short breaks; they may need to wind occasionally.
- Never leave the infant unattended with a bottle.
- Don't force the infant to finish a feed if they have had enough.
- Discard any leftover milk.

Lactation suppression

In some situations, mothers may need support and advice on suppressing lactation. NICE guidance (2021a) suggests discussion should include explanation on how breastmilk is produced, how long it will take to stop producing breastmilk and what happens when it stops. Mothers will also need the following self-help advice:

- To avoid stimulating the breast.
- Wearing a supportive bra.
- Use of ice packs.
- Pain relief.
- Expressing milk to ease engorgement.

Mothers should be advised when to seek further help and about prescribed medicines that suppress lactation if required. Depending on the situation, discussion about becoming a breastmilk donor may be appropriate.

Concluding comments

Although breastfeeding should be the norm for human infants, some infants or mothers are unable to, or choose not to, breastfeed. Healthcare professionals have a duty of care to ensure they can support these mothers to use alternative methods to meet the nutritional needs of their infants. For some, this is a temporary situation due to illness or separation. Therefore, careful consideration must be given to the method of providing nutrition so that it is not detrimental to later breastfeeding success. Unfortunately, many parents who choose to formula feed rather than breastfeed complain that they are not taught the technique of bottle feeding by healthcare professionals. This can have detrimental consequences for the health of the infant, and it is therefore imperative that midwives ensure that mothers are able to feed their infants confidently before being discharged from the hospital.

Reflective questions

- How do you decide what alternative method of feeding can be used for infants who are temporarily unable to breastfeed?
- What education do you provide for mothers, before discharge from hospital, who choose to formula feed their infants?
- How do you keep up to date on changes in formula milk and feeding equipment?

Resources

- Donor Milk Bank: Services Operation
  www.nice.org.uk/guidance/cg93

- NHS bottle-feeding guidance
  www.nhs.uk/conditions/baby/breastfeeding-and-bottle-feeding/

- PHS Formula Feeding www.healthscotland.com/uploads/documents/5523-__
  Formula%20feeding%20booklet-December2021-English.pdf

- United Kingdom Association of Milk Banks (UKAMB)
  www.ukamb.org

10 Introducing solid foods

Mothers need evidence-based advice and support to ensure that the timing of introducing solid food is appropriate and safe and does not result in any health problems. The introduction of solids (also referred to as complementary feeding or weaning) includes biting and chewing, which also develops the muscles required for speech development and tooth alignment. The WHO (2021a) recommends exclusive breastfeeding for the first six months of life and to continue alongside other foods for two years (see Chapter 1). This chapter aims to be a practical guide to introducing infants to solid food.

> - Learning outcomes
> - Introducing solid food
> - Baby-led weaning
> - Advice for parents on food types
> - Supplements
> - Concluding comments
> - Scenario
> - Further reading

Learning outcomes

By the end of this chapter, you will be able to:

- discuss the appropriate time to introduce solid foods;
- describe the signs of developmental readiness for the introduction of solid foods; and
- identify the appropriate foods to introduce during weaning.

Mapping to UNICEF Baby Friendly Initiative (BFI) Education learning outcomes (2019a)
By the end of the programme, students will:

Theme		Learning outcomes
Theme 1: Understand breastfeeding	2.	Understand the importance of human milk and breastfeeding to the health and wellbeing outcomes of mothers, babies and the wider family.

DOI: 10.4324/9781003282341-10

Theme		Learning outcomes
Theme 2: Support infant feeding	6.	Have the knowledge and skills to support mothers and babies to maximise breastmilk and breastfeeding, to continue to breastfeed for as long as they wish and to introduce solid foods at an appropriate time.
Theme 4: Managing the challenges	13.	Draw on their knowledge and understanding of the wider social, cultural and political influences which undermine breastfeeding, to promote, support and protect breastfeeding within their sphere of practice.
Theme 5: Communication	14.	Have an understanding of the principles of effective communication and current thinking around public health promotion strategies and approaches.

Introducing solid food

Introducing solid food before six months is not recommended because there is insufficient developmental readiness to cope with foods other than breast or formula milk. The aspects of developmental readiness relevant to introducing solid foods are:

- development of the infant's immune system;
- maturity of the gastrointestinal tract and kidneys;
- oral development and ability to chew; and
- hand-to-mouth coordination.

The WHO (2021a) recommends the gradual introduction of solid foods at six months for both breastfed infants and those who are formula fed. In addition, mothers need to be taught to recognise the signs to look out for that suggest their infants are ready to be weaned:

- They can maintain an upright sitting position on their own.
- They can co-ordinate their eyes, hand and mouth – they can look at the food, pick it up and put it in their mouths by themselves.
- They can swallow the food. If they are not ready will push their food back out of their mouths.

This should be followed by accurate advice and support on how to do this safely. Weaning should be a gradual process, while breastfeeding continues. As the infant adjusts to the changed regimen and new tastes and textures, another meal can be introduced. By the age of one year, the infant should be having three meals a day and eating a varied diet, supplemented with either breast or formula milk. Mothers should be encouraged to continue breastfeeding as long as the child requires. See www.nhs.uk/start4life for further information.

Key facts

The WHO (WHO, 2014a, 2021a) recommends that infants should be exclusively breastfed until the age of six months because:

- Breastmilk provides all the nutrients an infant requires for the first six months of life.
- Breastfeeding reduces the incidence of gastrointestinal, respiratory and ear infections.

- Breastfed infants are less likely to develop type 1 and 2 diabetes or become obese.
- The longer the mother breastfeeds, the less likely she is to develop premenopausal breast cancer and osteoporosis, and the quicker she will return to her pre-pregnancy weight.
- Menstruation and the return of fertility are delayed with exclusive breastfeeding.

The WHO (2021a) recommends two to three meals a day for infants six to eight months of age; from nine months, infants should be taking three meals a day. By this time, the infant should be eating a mixture of chopped, mashed and firmer finger foods such as fruit or bread sticks. From 12 months on, infants should be fitting in with family meals. (See www.nhs.uk/start4life/ for further information.)

Baby-led weaning

Rapley (2011) suggested that introducing infants to a variety of foods can be achieved by a common-sense approach she termed 'baby-led weaning'. Her theory was based on her observations during a small study in 2005 of five breastfed infants who were introduced to solids at four months of age (in line with recommendations at the time) and is based on the infants' development over the first year. At approximately six months, the digestive tract and immune system are ready for the introduction of other foods, and the infant is able to sit up, grab food and put it in the mouth and chew. However, Rapley urged caution about putting an exact time on weaning but instead providing the opportunities and allowing the baby to practice the skills when they show they are ready. She describes the concept as being part of shared mealtimes, part of a social occasion rather than led by hunger, the infant should be allowed to be curious and experiment with the food. Many parents worry about choking; www.nhs.uk offers safety and hygiene guidance. Fangupo *et al.* (2016) conducted a randomised controlled trial of 206 healthy infants allocated to a control or baby-led introduction to solids group to determine the impact of a baby-led approach to feeding on gagging and choking. Whilst they concluded that following a baby-led approach to feeding does not increase the risk of choking, they suggested that parents in both groups need more advice on safe foods and environments to avoid choking. Some parents have difficulty differentiating between gagging and choking; infants may gag when solid food is first introduced while learning to chew and swallow.

Safety guidance includes:

- The infant should be sitting upright (with the arms free).
- Only the infant should put food in her or his mouth.
- Do not leave infants alone with food.
- Remove stones from fruit.
- Do not give the infant nuts.
- Wash and peel fruit and vegetables.
- Hard foods like raw carrots and apples need to be cooked to soften them.
- Cut small, round foods, such as grapes, into small pieces.

Further information for parents can be found in the resources section at the end of this chapter.

Practice recommendations: gradual weaning

- Start slowly, offering the same food as the family that is easy to grasp and handle such as fist-sized soft fruit or vegetables.
- Once the infant is used to these tastes and textures, other healthy food can be introduced such as meat, fish and pasta.
- Allow food to cool, testing the temperature before giving it to the infant.
- Let the infant feed her- or himself as it is normal for infants to play with food to discover new textures and tastes; mothers must be prepared for the mess.
- Provide a variety of tastes and textures.
- Do not hurry the process of weaning; each infant will progress at an individual pace.
- Do not leave the infant alone while eating because of the risk of choking.
- Continue to observe nappies for urine output to avoid dehydration.

Rapley (2011) suggested that almost all food types can be introduced to the infant after six months of age alongside breastfeeding or formula feeding (see 'Advice for parents on food types' below). She recommended initially giving foods that can be easily cut up into hand-held sizes, long enough for some to protrude from the infant's fist, so the infant can hold it. She advises parents not to worry about the amount of food taken in the first few months, as breast or formula milk will provide adequate nutrition; early introduction to solid food should be fun and a learning experience. The following guidelines are adapted from Rapley's (2008) leaflet, *Baby-led Weaning*:

- Sit the infant upright facing a table.
- Offer food rather than feeding it to the infant.
- Start with food that is easy to pick up (hand-held size).
- Involve the infant at family mealtimes and, if suitable, offer the same food.
- Choose mealtimes when the infant is not tired.
- Continue breast or formula milk feeds but not necessarily at mealtimes.
- Offer water with meals.
- Do not hurry the process.
- Allow the infant to control the amount they want to eat.

Advice for parents on food types

The aim of weaning is to introduce infants to the variety of foods that the family eats. Similar to the *Infant Feeding Survey 2010* (McAndrew *et al.*, 2012), the *Scottish Maternal and Infant Feeding Survey* (SG, 2017) found that breakfast cereals, fruit and vegetables were most frequently given to infants. However, this survey found that those who lived in the most deprived areas were more likely to use commercial baby foods on a daily basis (Scottish Index of Multiple Deprivation [SIMD] 1: 38 per cent) than those in the least deprived areas (SIMD 5: 25 per cent). Those who lived in the most deprived areas were less likely to give fruit on a daily basis (SIMD 1: 61 per cent) than mothers in less deprived areas (SIMD 5: 76 per cent); vegetables, excluding potatoes or green leafy vegetables, on daily basis (SIMD 1: 44 per cent) than those in the least deprived areas (SIMD 5: 61 per cent) and dairy produce on daily basis (SIMD 1: 33 per cent) than mothers in the least deprived area (SIMD 5: 44 per cent). The *Infant Feeding Survey 2010* (McAndrew *et al.*, 2012) reported that mothers who introduced solid food after their infants were five months old were more likely to first introduce fruit and vegetables.

Boswell (2021) conducted a review of 29 studies which suggested baby-led weaning results in less food fussiness, increased food enjoyment and higher satiety responsiveness. Dogan *et al.* (2018) conducted a randomised controlled study with 280 healthy infants to assess growth, haematological parameters and iron intake at 12 months. They found those in the traditional spoon-feeding group were significantly heavier, but there were no differences in reported haematological parameters or iron intake.

Mothers should be given the following advice for preparing a healthy diet:

- Avoid foods high in salt, such as cheese, bacon, sausages and processed food not specifically prepared for infants, such as cereals and sauces, because the infant's renal system cannot process them.
- Avoid adding sugar to foods and drinks because it can cause tooth decay and encourages a 'sweet tooth'.
- Honey should be avoided in food for infants younger than one year old because of the risk of bacteria that could cause infant botulism. It also has the same issues as sugar (see earlier).
- Breastfed infants do not require additional drinks; however, formula-fed infants usually do and should be offered cooled boiled tap water or boiled bottled water with labels stating that it is safe for infants. Caution must be taken with bottled water as not all mineral water is suitable for infants.
- Fruit juice diluted (1:10) with cooled boiled water may be given to infants older than six months of age with a meal. However, because it contains sugar, which may cause tooth decay, it should be avoided at other times.
- Other drinks that contain sugars should be avoided to prevent tooth decay, particularly if given in a bottle, such as fizzy drinks, squash or flavoured milk. These additional drinks may also inhibit appetite and cause loose stools.
- Cow's, goat's and sheep's milk should not be given as a drink to infants younger than one year as they do not contain the required nutrients.
- Tea and coffee are not suitable drinks as they inhibit iron absorption.
  The website www.nhs.uk/start4life/weaning/what-to-feed-your-baby/ provides detailed advice and food recommendations commensurate with the infant's age.

If the mother decides to begin weaning before the recommended six months, it is suggested that this should not be before four months and food should be pureed to a smooth, thin consistency for example and served in a bowl (never in a bottle) for example pureed vegetables or fruit (PHS, 2022). Foods that may increase the risk of allergies should be avoided, such as:

- Bread, rusks and some cereals (gluten).
- Eggs.
- Fish and shellfish.
- Nuts and seeds.
- Soft and unpasteurised cheeses.

Supplements

It is recommended that infants should be given vitamin D drops from birth, unless receiving 500 ml or more of formula milk a day and that infants between the ages of six months and five years of age should be given supplements containing vitamins A, C and D unless feeding on formula to which the vitamins have been added. Infants on a vegan diet require vitamin B12 (DHSC, 2022).

Concluding comments

The decision of when to introduce solid food is a complex process for mothers and can be positively or negatively influenced by partners, family, friends and healthcare professionals, as well as socio-cultural traditions, as discussed in Chapter 1. Therefore, it is essential that healthcare professionals have the knowledge and skills to advise mothers confidently on how to recognise when their infants are ready for solid food, how to go about introducing it and what types of food to include in a healthy balanced diet.

Scenario

Khushi is a first-time breastfeeding mum. She has heard about baby-led weaning, but a relative has told her to start weaning using baby rice or mashed vegetables and to stop breastfeeding. Her five-month-old baby is gaining adequate weight and doesn't seem to like the mashed food.

- How would you advise Khushi at this stage and prepare her for weaning?

Further reading

- Public Health England: Starting Your Baby on Their First Solid Foods. www.nhs.uk/start4life/first-foods.
- Public Health England: Your baby's first solid food. www.nhs.uk/conditions/baby/weaning-and-feeding/babys-first-solid-foods/.
- Public Health Scotland: Fun Foods First. www.healthscotland.com/documents/303.aspx.

11 Ongoing support for breastfeeding mothers

- Learning outcomes
- Breastfeeding support
- Returning to work
- Sexual activity
- Family planning: lactational amenorrhoea method
- Breastfeeding during pregnancy: tandem nursing
- Relactation or induced lactation
- Concluding comments
- Reflective questions
- Resources

Breastfeeding mothers need ongoing support from professionals, their peers and society in general to continue breastfeeding for as long they would like to. Although many of the issues that influence duration of breastfeeding have been discussed throughout this book, this chapter will focus on particular issues such as accessing different types of support, returning to work and assisting mothers with relactation or induced lactation, family planning and breastfeeding during pregnancy.

Learning outcomes

By the end of this chapter, you will be able to:

- discuss the need for ongoing professional, social and peer support;
- advise mothers about both the legal and practical aspects of returning to work;
- assist mothers who have ceased breastfeeding to relactate or to induce lactation in those who wish to breastfeed; and
- provide advice about family planning, sexual activity and breastfeeding during pregnancy.

DOI: 10.4324/9781003282341-11

Mapping to UNICEF Baby Friendly Initiative (BFI) Education learning outcomes (2019a)

By the end of the programme, students will:

Theme		Learning outcomes
Theme 1: Understanding breastfeeding	1.	Have sufficient knowledge of anatomy of the breast and physiology of lactation to enable them to support mothers to successfully establish and maintain breastfeeding.
	2.	Understand the importance of human milk and breastfeeding to the health and wellbeing outcomes of mothers, babies and the wider family.
Theme 2: Support infant feeding	3.	Have an understanding of infant feeding culture within the UK and the various influences and constraints which impact on women's infant feeding decisions.
	6.	Have the knowledge and skills to support mothers and babies to maximise breastmilk and breastfeeding, to continue to breastfeed for as long as they wish and to introduce solid foods at an appropriate time.
Theme 4: Manage the challenges	13.	Draw on their knowledge and understanding of the wider social, cultural and political influences which undermine breastfeeding, to promote, support and protect breastfeeding within their sphere of practice.
Theme 5: Promote positive communication	14.	Have an understanding of the principles of effective communication and current thinking around public health promotion strategies and approaches.
	15.	Be able to apply their knowledge of effective communication to initiate sensitive, compassionate, mother-centred conversations with pregnant women and new mothers.

It is clear throughout this book that the evidence supports the fact that breastmilk is the best form of nutrition for human infants and has positive health benefits for both mother and infant, and the longer an infant is breastfed, the greater the benefits are. The *Infant Feeding Survey 2010* (McAndrew *et al.*, 2012) demonstrated that the breastfeeding initiation rates for the UK increased compared with the *Infant Feeding Survey 2005* (Bolling *et al.*, 2007): from 78 to 83 per cent in England, 70 to 74 per cent in Scotland, 67 to 71 per cent in Wales and 63 to 64 per cent in Northern Ireland. However, the pattern for a rapid decline over the first week continued from 81 per cent to 69 per cent – 55 per cent at six weeks postpartum, and 34 per cent at six months. Since the cessation of the *Infant Feeding Survey*, it is more difficult to get a clear picture across the UK due to different methodologies in collating data. The *Scottish Maternal and Infant Nutrition Survey* (SG, 2017), however, found:

- Three-quarters of respondents to both postnatal surveys had 'ever' breastfed and/or expressed milk for their new baby (75 per cent of the 8–12-week survey and 76 per cent of the 8–12-month survey).
- More than two-thirds of all respondents (69 per cent) were giving breastmilk to their babies when they left the maternity unit.

- Three-quarters of respondents (75 per cent) who had stopped giving breastmilk reported that they would have liked to have given breastmilk for longer.

The WHO target for 2015 was not achieved, and breastfeeding rates continue to be a long way from meeting the WHO 2025 (2014a) recommendation for 50 per cent exclusive breastfeeding at six months. The updated global targets for 2030 are 70 per cent for initiation in the first hour, 70 per cent for exclusive breastfeeding, 80 per cent at one year, and 60 per cent at two years (WHO/UNICEF, 2021).

Similar to Bolling *et al.* (2007) and McAndrew *et al.* (2012), the *Scottish Maternal and Infant Nutrition Survey* (SG, 2017) identified older mothers, first-time mothers and those who lived in the least deprived areas were more likely to have ever breastfed and/or expressed breastmilk for their baby. There is limited information on ethnic groups from this study as 92–94 per cent of respondents indicated that 'white' best described their ethnic group.

McInnes and Chambers highlighted that, in general, mothers reported that 'a lack of breastfeeding knowledge acted as a barrier to their receiving and accepting postnatal support' (2008b, p. 423). This was supported by O'Brien *et al.* (2009), who identified that the strategies mothers used to successfully breastfeed included increasing breastfeeding knowledge, goal setting and challenging unhelpful beliefs. Gavine *et al.* (2022) conducted a systematic review of 116 randomised controlled studies to examine breastfeeding support interventions. They suggest extra organised support helps mothers to breastfeed for longer, particularly if four to eight visits are scheduled. They did not find a difference in who provided the support (professional or non-professional) or how it was provided (face to face, digital, phone) as this may be dependent on the setting and population group. Furthermore, they stated it is probable that fewer mothers stop breastfeeding at four to six weeks and three to four months. Regan and Brown (2019) interviewed 14 mothers to explore their experiences breastfeeding and motivations and experiences of accessing online support. They suggested that due to the lack of investment in breastfeeding, mothers were more frequently using online support groups that could lead to seeking face-to-face support. Participants said the support received often helped them continue to breastfeed; however, some groups could have very polarised views on infant feeding or were not moderated, leading to sharing of misinformation. Despite this, participants found these groups provided a safe space where they valued the emotional support from others with similar experiences.

However, as demonstrated throughout this book, the factors that influence the initiation and duration of breastfeeding come from international, national and regional levels as well as from the individual (Dyson *et al.*, 2006). Table 11.1 summarises these issues.

Breastfeeding support

Professional support

McInnes and Chambers (2008b) conducted a review of qualitative literature to produce a synthesis of mothers' and healthcare professionals' experiences and perceptions of breastfeeding support. They concluded that mothers did not receive the support they wanted from healthcare professionals and that healthcare professionals were not the main source of postnatal support; instead, social support was considered to be of greater value. Both mothers and professionals reported that poor staffing levels in postnatal wards resulted in conflicting advice and in a lack of information and support. They suggest that conflicting advice and poor techniques may be results of a lack of education and training and recommend practical skills training, updates, mentoring and assessment for staff, as well

Table 11.1 Examples of factors (often interrelated) that influence infant feeding at international, national, regional and individual levels

International and national factors	National and regional factors	Individual factors – amenable to medium- to long-term change at the macro socio-economic level	Individual factors influencing decision to breastfeed – amenable to change in the short term at the micro socio-economic level	Individual factors influencing a woman's decision to stop breastfeeding before she wishes – amenable to change in the short term at the micro level
Globalisation of formula feeding in developed countries promulgated by commercial interests	Lack of importance or understanding of breastfeeding in the organisation of health services; embedded practices or routines that interfere with successful breastfeeding	Maternal age – younger mothers are less likely to breastfeed	Attitudes of partner, mother and peer group	Mother's or health professionals' or family's perception of 'insufficient milk'
Cultural shift to regimented feeding patterns and growth of monitoring based on formula-feeding regimens	Lack of appropriate education and training for health and related professionals	Maternal education – breastfeeding rates are lowest among those who left school at 16 or less	Social support provided by woman's partner, family and friends	Painful breasts and nipples; baby would not suck or 'rejected the breast'
Increase in work opportunities for women without supportive childcare or feeding facilities	Lack of integration across sectors – acute, community, social services, voluntary	Socio-economic status of mother (and partner) – breastfeeding rates become lower for lower socio-economic groups	Loss of collective knowledge and experience of breastfeeding in the community, resulting in a lack of confidence in breastfeeding	Breastfeeding takes too long or is tiring
Media portrayal of bottle feeding as the norm and as safe	Lack of supportive environments outside the home and in the workplace	Marital status; ethnicity – cultural tendency for White women to choose not to breastfeed	Whether mothers were breastfed themselves as babies	Mother or baby is ill; difficult to judge how much baby has drunk
Increased media portrayal of women's breasts as symbols of sexuality	Lack of breastfeeding education in schools	Biomedical factors (parity, method of delivery, infant health)	Embarrassment about, difficulty in, or perceived unacceptability of breastfeeding in public, both in and outside the home, especially for younger mothers	Baby can't be fed by others
Lack of full implementation of WHO Code of Marketing of Breastmilk Substitutes		Return to work before the baby is four months old	Difficulty of involving others, especially partner, in feeding; perceived inconvenience of breastfeeding and anxiety about total dependence of the baby on the mother	

as the need to include interpersonal and communication skills. Building a therapeutic relationship is important when providing support for breastfeeding, as mothers are more receptive if they feel comfortable asking questions and do not feel judged. Practical and consistent advice and information, encouragement and emotional support are crucial elements in developing this relationship, as is continuity of care or carers where possible. These findings are supported by Blixt *et al.* (2019), who conducted an exploratory study asking women what advice they would give professionals who support breastfeeding mothers. They identified the importance of evidence-based support provided in a sensitive and individual way which would increase self-confidence and promote a positive experience of breastfeeding.

Social support

Mothers are more likely to breastfeed if they have a supportive social network. According to McInnes and Chambers (2008b, p. 422), support with breastfeeding can be split into three categories:

Practical	Housework, caring for other children
Information	Knowledge of breastfeeding
Emotional	Empathy, approval, praise, feeling nurtured

Social support depends on the societal norms for infant feeding and the knowledge, views and beliefs of family and friends. A supportive family network is considered essential for some mothers to overcome challenges they may face. Mothers also value support from those they perceive as 'role models' or who have had experience of breastfeeding, often their own mothers.

Although McInnes and Chambers (2008b) suggest that mothers value support from those with experience of breastfeeding, fathers also play an import ant role. When their attitude was positive towards breastfeeding, fathers were able to provide practical, physical and emotional support in the decision to breastfeed as well as to support continuation (Sheriff *et al.*, 2009). Sheriff *et al.* (2014, p. 21) conducted a concept analysis and systematic literature review resulting in the identification of five essential attributes of father support:

- Knowledge about breastfeeding.
- Positive attitude to breastfeeding.
- Involvement in the decision-making process.
- Practical support.
- Emotional support.

However, some men lack knowledge about breastfeeding and believe it will interfere with their relationship, particularly with regard to sex (Hewitt, 2008). In Western culture, breasts are often portrayed as sexual objects and often discussed as the 'man's property' (Dickens, 2008).

Sihota *et al.* (2019) undertook a scoping of 18 studies to explore the experiences, roles and needs of fathers of breastfed babies. They highlighted the need for antenatal education and support tailored for fathers and recognising them as fundamental to the breastfeeding triad would support the promotion of breastfeeding. Wang *et al.* (2018) also found that mothers tend to breastfeed for longer if they believe the father prefers exclusive breastfeeding.

It is clear that family and friends also need to be educated about the benefits of breastfeeding and the risks of formula feeding so they can provide adequate support for breastfeeding mothers. Many hospitals and community areas have developed innovative ways of doing this, from inviting fathers and prospective grandparents to breastfeeding classes, to developing posters to inform fathers of the benefits (Hewitt, 2008) and breastfeeding campaigns. However, if the social network is unsupportive, breastfeeding can be easily undermined, and mothers may feel pressurised into stopping breastfeeding or develop a lack of confidence in their ability. Some will seek out other forms of social support, such as peer support groups, and will join voluntary organisations. This was highlighted as particularly important when information was not forthcoming from healthcare professionals or they were unable to help solve problems (McInnes and Chambers, 2008b).

Today more mothers are looking for support through social media, such as Facebook groups. Bridges (2016) explored the experiences of mothers using a closed Facebook site attached to the Australian Breastfeeding Association and how they sought and shared information. Instead of being a threat to current services, it was found to provide an immediate, complementary and 'value-added' service. Herron *et al.* (2015) also explored online breastfeeding support and found it to be a cost-effective resource when mothers benefited from the opportunity 'to query, ponder, discuss, debate and rant about breastfeeding issues'. Approximately half of those who accessed an online resource to initiate or maintain breastfeeding did so for weeks or months.

Peer support

Peer support programmes were originally set up in areas of deprivation with poor breastfeeding rates. They either provide support on a one-to-one basis or to groups of women. The aim of these programmes is to improve breastfeeding rates in local communities by putting mothers in touch with other women with breastfeeding experience who can provide support, encouragement and practical advice. The intention is that a peer supporter will have similar demographic characteristics and understanding of the cultural expectations within the local area. Peer supporters receive training but are encouraged to refer complex problems to healthcare professionals. However, this training appears to vary across the UK. Thomson and Crossland (2019) highlighted the criticism that breastfeeding peer support interventions lacked theoretical underpinning. They used the Behavioural Change Wheel to structure an evaluation on how a peer support programme in Northwest England had been operationalised. Whilst they identified gaps and areas for development, they also found the service enhanced mothers' capability, motivation and opportunities to breastfeed. Ingram *et al.* (2020) developed an assets-based approach underpinned by change theory available to mothers whether they intended to breast of formula feed. The programme reported higher initiation of breastfeeding and continuation at eight weeks and six months compared to usual care.

Islam (2016) conducted a local evaluation in two deprived areas of London where uptake of peer support programmes was poor. Islam reported that these 'hard to reach' women had insurmountable barriers to initiating and sustaining breastfeeding. Some women had never heard of peer support, others reported it as 'a journey into the unknown' and one they were not prepared to take. In conclusion, she recommends peer supporters need to work more closely with health visitors and to be involved early during the antenatal period.

A number of studies have been carried out since the introduction of peer supporters, demonstrating varying success of programmes. Kaunonen *et al.* (2012) conducted a systematic review to describe peer support interventions during pregnancy and the postnatal period. They found that individual support and education were commonly used and that a combination of professional and peer support by trained peer supporters was most effective, but it had to be continuous. This is supported by Gavine *et al.* (2022), who also found that peer support had a positive impact on breastfeeding outcomes but that it should be offered on a scheduled basis.

Activity

- Find out what peer support programmes are available in your area and what the mechanism for referral is. How do women know about them?
- How do you educate family and friends about breastfeeding to support breastfeeding mothers?

Other support organisations

Midwives and other healthcare professionals should be familiar with the national and local breastfeeding support organisations. Some examples of such organisations are:

- Association of Breastfeeding Mothers (www.abm.me.uk)

  This was established in 1980 by mothers to give other mothers support and accurate information about breastfeeding.

- La Leche League (www.laleche.org.uk)

  The La Leche League was formed in 1956 by seven mothers who wanted to support breastfeeding friends. Today they have branches in over 60 countries, and their aim remains the same: to offer accurate mother-to-mother breastfeeding support. The organisation is predominantly run by volunteers who lead local groups. As well as providing training for breastfeeding supporters, La Leche publishes information for mothers and healthcare professionals; many are familiar with *The Breastfeeding Answer Book*, which is a valuable resource in many healthcare settings.

- National Childbirth Trust (www.nct.org.uk)

  The National Childbirth Trust is a UK organisation and was formed in 1956. Volunteers provide support for breastfeeding mothers through training and education for parents, counsellors and health professionals.

- Breastfeeding Network (www.breastfeedingnetwork.org.uk)

  The Breastfeeding Network is a recognised Scottish charity. Its aim is to promote breastfeeding, disseminate accurate, evidence-based information to parents and health professionals, and set standards for breastfeeding support.

- UNICEF BFI (www.unicef.org.uk/babyfriendly)

    The UNICEF BFI predominantly promotes best practice for breastfeeding mothers within healthcare and higher education settings and offers assessment and accreditation to acknowledge that these institutions achieve high standards. It also provides information for parents; however, it is unable to offer this on an individual basis.

Activity

There are numerous voluntary organisations throughout the UK to support breastfeeding mothers.

- Do you know the groups in your area of practice?
- Prepare a list of local groups that you can give to mothers in your care.

Returning to work

Many mothers want to continue breastfeeding after they return to work but often perceive this as a barrier to continuing breastfeeding. The benefits of continuing breastfeeding in line with the WHO recommendations (exclusive breastfeeding for six months and to continue for up to two years) for mothers and infants are well known, but there are also benefits for employers. NHS Health Scotland (2016, p. 14) states that these are:

- Reduced parental absence as breastfed infants are less likely to be ill compared to formula-fed infants.
- Higher rate of return to work of valued employees.
- Increased staff morale and loyalty.
- Lower recruitment and training costs.
- Recruitment incentives.

Legislation

Employers are legally bound to facilitate continued breastfeeding outside normal break times. It is best if this is planned in advance and employers are notified in writing before the mother returns to work so that preparations can be made. The following legislation protects breastfeeding mothers.

Management of Health and Safety at Work Regulations of 1999
(2000 Northern Ireland) and Employment Rights Act of 2002

The employer has a duty to carry out a risk assessment to assess whether working conditions are a risk to the health of the breastfeeding mother or infant. Some employers may not appreciate the dangers of not breastfeeding, and therefore it may be helpful if the mother provides them with some literature.

    If a risk is identified, it is the employer's responsibility to reduce the risk (see www.hse.gov.uk/mothers/employer/risk-assessment.htm). This may include temporarily adjusting the mother's working conditions and/or hours of work; if that is not possible, offering her suitable alternative work (at the same rate of pay) (Employment Rights Act, 1996); or if not possible suspending her from work on paid leave for as long as necessary to protect her health and safety and that of her child. If working hours need to be changed, for example, to avoid night shifts, this request can be supported by a medical certificate from the GP.

Workplace (Health, Safety and Welfare) Regulations of 1992

The Workplace Regulations require employers to provide suitable rest facilities for workers who are pregnant or breastfeeding. Ideally, these should be private, have hand-washing facilities and include facilities for the storage of breastmilk.

Equality Act of 2010

A breach of the Management of Health and Safety at Work Regulations may be unlawful under the Equality Act, depending on the circumstances.

EU Council Directive 92/85/EEC

This directive is for those working in the public sector. If the employee's work causes problems with breastfeeding, the employer must change the working conditions and/or hours for as long as she is breastfeeding.

Sex Discrimination Act of 1975 (1976 Northern Ireland)

If a woman is required to work particular hours without justification or has unfavourable conditions for breastfeeding, it can be considered as direct discrimination.

Maternity Leave and Parental Rights of 2003

Statutory maternity leave is for 52 weeks. This is 26 weeks of ordinary maternity leave (when a mother is entitled to all her contractual rights such as annual leave) and 26 of extra maternity leave (partially paid).

Shared Parental Leave (SPL) can be taken in three separate blocks, but employers must have at least eight weeks' notice. Parents can work up to 20 days while taking SPL without ending it. These are called Shared Parental Leave in Touch (SPLIT) and are in addition to ten Keeping in Touch (KIT) days, which are optional (www.gov.uk/employee-rights-when-on-leave).

Practicalities of returning to work

Mothers may choose different options for providing their infants with breastmilk while they are at work:

- Express breastmilk and leave it for a carer to give the infant. This may mean expressing milk during working hours, which will also maintain lactation and prevent the breasts becoming overfull.

- Use childcare facilities near the workplace so they can either breastfeed during the day or immediately before or after work.
- Negotiate shorter or flexible work hours.

The Health and Safety Executive has produced a range of useful resources for new and expectant mothers who work, which can be found at www.hse.gov.uk/mothers.

Expressing milk at work

Mothers should not be expected to express milk in the toilet or other unsuitable environment. A clean, warm and comfortable room should be made available with hand-washing facilities and somewhere to store equipment. If a fridge is not available, breastmilk should be stored in a cool bag. Depending on facilities, a mother may use a hand or electric pump or hand express. See Chapter 4 for further details about expressing and storing breastmilk.

Sexual activity

Some women resume sexual activity before the postpartum examination at six weeks. It is therefore important that issues related to sexual activity and conception are addressed earlier than this. For others, there may be a delay due to fatigue, a decrease in sexual desire, or vaginal dryness leading to dyspareunia due to a reduction in levels of oestrogen and androgens (Khajehei *et al.*, 2015). Some mothers report milk ejection during sexual activity and increased vaginal dryness. If the milk ejection is a problem for the couple, the mother can wear a bra with breast pads. Many women find it difficult to discuss sexual problems due to embarrassment, so this should be raised for discussion in a sensitive way.

Family planning: lactational amenorrhoea method

The lactational amenorrhoea method (LAM) is a natural method of family planning. During breastfeeding, prolactin inhibits the release of gonadotropin-releasing hormone and levels of oestrogen and progesterone are reduced, inhibiting ovulation. It is thought that LAM is 98 per cent effective in the first six months postpartum; however, it is reliant on exclusive and regular breastfeeding and staying amenorrhoeic (no vaginal blood loss for at least ten days after postpartum bleeding) (Van der Wijden and Manion, 2015).

If these factors do not apply, the mother should not rely on breastfeeding alone as a method of contraception and will require advice on appropriate alternative contraceptives. An intrauterine device or the progesterone-only contraceptive pill may be used when breastfeeding, but the combined oestrogen and progesterone pill must be avoided because it reduces the milk supply.

Breastfeeding during pregnancy: tandem nursing

Some mothers become pregnant while breastfeeding and may express concerns that they will have to wean the infant from the breast despite wanting to continue breastfeeding. Many mothers are misinformed and told they will have to stop breastfeeding; however, there is no danger to the fetus, and breastfeeding can continue in most cases. Advice should be sought if the mother has had a previous miscarriage or preterm birth or experiences bleeding. There is no evidence to suggest that the oxytocin released during breastfeeding will cause the uterus to contract, as oxytocin receptors in the uterus are inhibited until near term. Mothers need support and advice regarding taking adequate rest and appropriate diet, given the additional demands on them both physically and psychologically. Some mothers complain of tender nipples during pregnancy, and therefore attention to position and attachment is required.

Sinkiewicz-Darol *et al.* (2021) examined milk samples from 13 mothers who were tandem feeding and found that the breastmilk meets the needs of both the children. Fat content, energy value and protein concentration were higher, while carbohydrate content remained the same.

Once the new infant is born, he or she should be fed first because an adequate supply of colostrum is essential for newborns, and the older infant is getting nutrition from other sources at this point.

Relactation or induced lactation

Relactation or induced lactation is the stimulation of the breast to lactate to breastfeed an infant when pregnancy has been absent or to re-stimulate lactation following cessation of breastfeeding. Some mothers may have a reduced milk supply or have discontinued breastfeeding for a variety of reasons and regret the decision. It is important that healthcare professionals are aware that this situation is reversible and develop the skills to enable the mothers to lactate and commence or recommence breastfeeding.

The aim is to trigger the release of prolactin and oxytocin to commence milk production; however, for some mothers, not all the prolactin receptors will have been primed initially, and therefore full production may not be possible. Inducing lactation requires great commitment, and therefore the mother should be very motivated and made aware that it may take a few weeks to establish adequate milk production. Skilled help and support from professionals are required to teach the skills needed to induce lactation and to give the mother confidence in her ability to do so on a day-to-day basis. She will also need support from her family and friends so the process is not undermined. Putting her in contact with other mothers who have relactated or induced lactation may be helpful. When Lommens *et al.* (2013) asked mothers who chose to relactate about their experiences and found mothers focused on the emotional aspects of relactation rather than the physical process.

Before induced lactation commences, a full history must be taken as to why the mother had a poor milk supply or why she discontinued breastfeeding to ensure that there are no factors that may continue to inhibit milk production, such as prolonged separation from the infant, supplementary feeding, use of teats or dummies, smoking, the combined contraceptive pill or medical reasons. Once the reason is identified, this must be rectified, when possible, before continuing the process.

The process of induced lactation

As identified by Mohd Hassan *et al.* (2021), there is limited evidence around induced lactation. They conducted a review of the literature over the past 60 years and were only able to find 17 articles of 50 that included women's experiences. They found enablers to successful induced lactation could be psychosocial or technical-pharmacological and non-pharmacological methods such as breast stimulation. Challenges include internal and external factors such as personal behaviour and environmental factors including support. The WHO (1998b) suggests there are two essential requirements for inducing lactation: 'a strong desire by the mother or foster mother to feed the infant, and stimulation of the nipple'.

Maximum stimulation of the nipple and breast can be achieved by the following techniques:

- There should be long periods of uninterrupted skin-to-skin contact and access to the breast. Co-bathing is one way of providing a comfortable and relaxing environment.
- Position and attachment should be retaught, along with recognising feeding cues.
- Breastfeed and/or express milk 8–12 times per day. Include night times when there is an increased production of prolactin.
- Practice breast compression if the milk flow is slow.
- Avoid artificial teats and dummies.
- Use of a breastfeeding supplementer (see Chapter 9) during breastfeeding may encourage the infant to suckle when the milk supply is poor.

While the mother is establishing her milk supply, it is important that the infant's nutritional needs are met. If expressed breastmilk is available, this should be given following a breastfeed; however, this may not be available for all infants, and they may require formula milk. As it is important to avoid teats, this can be given by cup or spoon. The infant should be closely observed to ensure their nutritional needs are being met by assessing wet nappies and stool as well as weight gain.

If these methods are not effective, pharmacological methods (galactagogues such as domperidone or metoclopramide) or herbal remedies (such as fenugreek, garlic or fennel) may be tried, but further research is required to assess their effectiveness when milk production has ceased altogether (WHO, 1998b).

Concluding comments

Professional, social and peer support is an important element in providing mothers with help and information to enable them to continue to breastfeed for as long as they want to. To do this, healthcare professionals must know of and share national and local support for breastfeeding with mothers and refer as appropriate. It is also important that there is continued cooperation between healthcare staff, breastfeeding support groups and the local community.

To ensure community support is effective, healthcare professionals must be educated and develop the knowledge and skills required to be able to support and advise mothers with practical and useful information as well as provide evidence-based information for fathers, family and friends. How they develop this knowledge and skill is the focus of the following chapter.

Reflective questions

1　What models of support are offered in your areas?
2　When do you inform women about peer support programmes?
3　Do you use a model to encourage fathers to promote and support breastfeeding?

4 How is information disseminated to fathers, families and friends in your area of practice?

5 What follow-up mechanisms are in place for breastfeeding mothers in the community to assist them to continue to breastfeed exclusively until their infants are six months old?

Resources

- HSE: *Protecting pregnant workers and new mothers*
  www.hse.gov.uk/mothers

- La Leche League
  www.laleche.org.uk

- NHS UK: *Breastfeeding and work*
  www.nhs.uk/conditions/baby/breastfeeding-and-bottle-feeding/breastfeeding-and-lifestyle/back-to-work/

- UNICEF Baby Friendly Initiative
  www.unicef.org.uk/babyfriendly/

12 Developing knowledge and skills to support breastfeeding mothers

- Learning outcomes
- Informed choice
- Communication skills
- Trauma-informed practice
- Learning about breastfeeding
- Concluding comments
- Reflective questions

To support and advise breastfeeding mothers effectively, it is essential that midwives, health visitors and other healthcare professionals have the knowledge and skills to do this. The Nursing and Midwifery Council's professional standards, 'The Code', stipulates that nurses, midwives and health visitors must practice effectively and:

- practice in line with the best available evidence;
- communicate clearly;
- work cooperatively;
- share skills, knowledge and experience for the benefit both of people receiving care and colleagues;
- keep clear and accurate records relevant to the practice; and
- be accountable for decisions to delegate tasks and duties to other people.

(NMC, 2015, pp. 10–14)

This chapter discusses the essential skills required by healthcare professionals to enable them to provide mothers and their families with accurate information and skilled support, so that they can make informed choices, for example communication skills, reflective practice and evidence-based practice. In addition, a trauma-informed approach is explored.

Learning outcomes

By the end of this chapter, you will be able to:

- understand what influences mothers in their infant feeding choices;
- demonstrate effective communication and teaching skills; and

DOI: 10.4324/9781003282341-12

- reflect on the knowledge and skills required to promote, protect and support breast-feeding and demonstrate how they can be achieved.

Mapping to UNICEF Baby Friendly Initiative (BFI) Education learning outcomes (2019a)

By the end of the programme, students will:

Theme		Learning outcomes
Theme 5: Promote positive communication	14.	Have an understanding of the principles of effective communication and current thinking around public health promotion strategies and approaches.
	15.	Be able to apply their knowledge of effective communication to initiate sensitive, compassionate, mother-centred conversations with pregnant women and new mothers.
	16.	Have the knowledge and skills to access the evidence-based information that underpins infant feeding practice and know how to keep up-to-date (e.g. e-alerts, research summaries).

Informed choice

To enable women to make informed choices about their care, healthcare professionals must 'provide accessible, evidence-based information in a balanced and non-judgemental manner and then respect whatever option is chosen' (Adamson, 2004, p. 587). This can sometimes be difficult for healthcare professionals, who are aware of the evidence to support breastfeeding and at times have difficulty understanding why mothers make the choices they do. Mothers studied have been found to have made their choices mainly based on personal or vicarious experience (Dykes, 2003; Battersby, 2014), and professionals must be able to understand and predict this. Similar to the *Infant Feeding Survey 2010* (McAndrew *et al.*, 2012), the *Scottish Maternal and Infant Nutrition Survey* (SG, 2017) identified that most respondents who were planning to use formula instead of breastfeeding found discussion with health professionals helpful but rarely influenced their decision. This further highlights the important role of the healthcare practitioner in providing clear, practical information about the benefits of breastfeeding in terms all mothers can understand and in being able to answer any questions, thereby dispelling any myths. However, despite being provided with information on the benefits of breast-feeding, many mothers will still choose to formula feed either immediately after birth or at some point later on. It is important that this decision is respected and mothers are given the support and advice to do this correctly and safely (see Chapter 9).

It is also important to consider the impact healthcare professionals' personal views and experience has on their ability to promote and support breastfeeding. Marks and O'Connor (2015) conducted a qualitative study of 51 healthcare practitioners to explore this issue. Although they uncovered a range of attitudes, the practitioners were in agreement that breastfeeding was better than formula feeding. Nevertheless, some participants felt a powerlessness and pessimism due to the impact of other influences (family and friends) and perceived their influence to be minimal. Some also reported the fine line between breastfeeding promotion and coercion due to 'over-zealous' promotion and the moral judgment inherent in it. To address this, Marks and O'Connor (2015, p. 861) recommended staff training that raises the awareness of psychological processes that can have an impact on breastfeeding promotion behaviour.

Communication skills

Many mothers perceive healthcare professionals as too busy to spend time with them, and therefore it is important to create an environment that promotes a relaxed and un-rushed atmosphere to encourage the physiology of lactation. Communication should not only be about the exchange or transfer of information but also about how it contributes to the therapeutic relationship – getting to know the mother and what she wants from the situation. Good communication skills enable healthcare professionals to build relationships and provide emotional support for mothers and give clear, accurate and relevant information to empower mothers to breastfeed with confidence and to carry out effective breastfeeding assessments. Poor communication can lead to a mother experiencing a loss of control over her situation, stress, anxiety and sometimes misunderstanding or conflicting advice, which ultimately leads to lack of support. As discussed in Chapter 2, stress and anxiety can have a profound effect on the physiology of lactation and undermine a mother's confidence in her ability to breastfeed.

Communication of any message is a complex process and takes verbal, non-verbal and symbolic forms. For a message to be transferred effectively, there must be a shared understanding of the content and structure of the message, which involves appreciation of attitudes, knowledge, social and cultural ideas that both the sender and receiver of the message possess. Often healthcare professionals assume that others understand professional terminology and abbreviations and take it for granted that they have prior understanding of the context of the message. A useful tool often used to explain the processes of communication in nursing and midwifery is based on Aristotle's theory of the requirements for effective communication, 'Speaker – Subject – Audience', which has been further developed by many writers such as Shannon and Weaver in 1949 and Berlo in the 1960s. (See Januszewski, 2001 for details of various communication models.) The model in Figure 12.1 is based on these ideas.

- Sender

  The sender is the person or persons (organisation) who begin the communication process and are responsible for encoding or translating the message. This may be influenced by the sender's attitude, knowledge and social and cultural experiences.

- Transmitter

  The content of the message is encoded or translated and structured using symbols such as language, literature, pictures or other non-verbal cues, etc. It is critical at this point that these symbols can be understood by the receiver for communication to be effective.

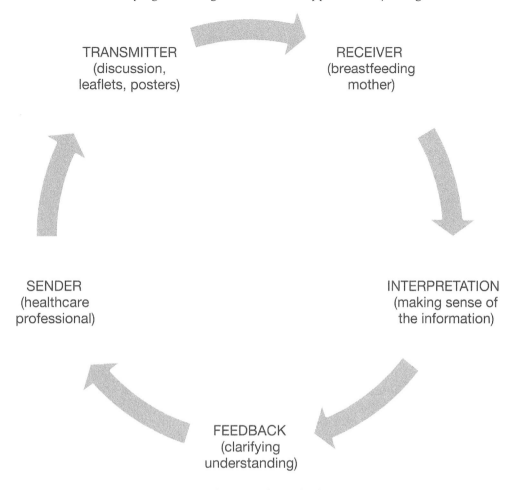

Figure 12.1 Communication processes: discussing breastfeeding

- Receiver

  The person receives the message through the senses, such as hearing, seeing, touching or tasting, and begins the process of decoding or interpretation.

- Interpretation

  Interpretation takes place using the same processes that the sender used to construct the message, attitude, knowledge and social and cultural experiences to make sense of the message.

- Feedback

  Berlo (1960) suggested that the communication process was incomplete until feedback from the receiver was received by the sender and the sender had in turn responded. The aim is to clarify that shared understanding has taken place.

Barriers to good communication

Between transmission and receiving, there can be interference leading to misunderstanding or the message never being received. This can be caused by the following:

- *Non-verbal cues*: negative body language – facial expressions, posture or poor eye contact.
- *Language*: technical terminology, too much information, language barriers, and level and tone of voice.
- *Attitude*: cultural and social norms, values and rules, pre-conceived ideas, prejudice and previous experience.
- *Individual aspects*: health and emotional status and cognitive skills.
- *Environment*: appropriateness to message – privacy, noise or distraction.

Lubbers (1990) suggested that the six most important skills for communication are:

- Listening.
- Relationship-building.
- Instructing.
- Motivation.
- Exchanging information.
- Giving feedback.

It could be argued that emotional intelligence could be added to this list. The main components of emotional intelligence are understanding yourself and understanding others through self-awareness, social awareness, self-management and social skills, all of which are essential for good communication processes.

It is important that women are given appropriate information to make informed choices. Part of this is ensuring that mothers receive unbiased information that is based on evidence. Every mother will perceive her breastfeeding experience differently, and these experiences should not be undermined or judged by the healthcare professional. Nor should it be assumed that she has the knowledge she needs to breastfeed successfully even if she has had previous experience.

UNICEF UK BFI have strengthened their focus on communication skills and developed a series on having meaningful conversations with mothers by using signature sheets as an aid memoir. They also become part of the mother's record so they can be shared and reviewed by all staff involved in care. The focus of this series is building relationships and trust by moving the emphasis from a directional approach (a tick box approach to transmitting information) to a guiding approach (conversation involving active listening, providing information and alternatives) (UNICEF UK BFI, n.d.; Rollnick *et al.*, 2008).

There is evidence that pregnant women and new mothers have increased right brain dominance (intuitive), leading to greater sensitivity to non-verbal communication and less receptivity to large amounts of information. UNICEF UK BFI (n.d., p. 5) provide the following recommendations to keep conversations woman-centred:

- Agree on an agenda.
- Ask open questions.

- Listen actively.
- Reflect back.
- Find out and build on information she knows.
- Show empathy.
- Remain neutral.
- Don't collude.

Activity

Reflect on a recent experience where you were trying to convey information to a breastfeeding mother.

- Did the communication process remain intact?
- Did she understand the message and give you feedback to clarify a shared understanding?
- If not, what do you think went wrong and how would you change things in the future?
- How did you gauge if the process was effective?

The NMC Standards of Proficiency for Midwives (2019, pp. 33–34), Domain 6, identifies the key 'skills required when communicating with women, their partners and families, and colleagues that take account of women's needs, views, preferences, and decisions' and 'approaches for building relationships and sharing information with women, their partners and families that ensures that women's needs, views, preferences, and decisions can be supported in all circumstances' (Table 12.1). In addition, Annexe A of the Future Nurse: Standards of Proficiency for Registered Nurses (NMC, 2018) includes guidance on the communication and relationship management skills that registered nurses must be able to demonstrate.

The focus of Domain 6 (NMC, 2019) is on person-centred care, taking account of the woman's needs, views and preferences and adapting to meet specific needs. Some people have very specific communication needs. These include hearing, vision and other physical, mental and cognitive abilities, as well as language and any requirement for an interpreter. Effective communication ensures mothers are actively involved and as required, reasonable adjustments are made to share information in an understandable way.

Learning disability

NHS UK (2022) describe learning disability as being different for each individual and can affect the way people learn new things, particularly understanding new information and learning some skills. Autism can affect how people communicate and interact with others and experience the world around them. Sometimes sensory sensitivity can be an issue and can be confused with breastfeeding aversion, but this will vary with individuals. Mothers with learning disabilities can also have complex needs resulting from other issues such as discrimination and poor self-esteem. Whilst the exact number of the UK population with

Table 12.1 NMC Standards of Proficiency for Midwives (2019, pp. 33–34)

Domain 6: Communication, sharing information and relationship management

6.1	demonstrate the ability to use evidence-based communication skills when communicating and sharing information with the woman, newborn infants and families that takes account of the woman's needs, views, preferences, and decisions, and the needs of the newborn infant
6.1.1	actively listen, recognise and respond to verbal and non-verbal cues
6.1.2	use prompts and positive verbal and non-verbal reinforcement
6.1.3	use appropriate non-verbal communication techniques including touch, eye contact, and respecting personal space
6.1.4	make appropriate use of respectful, caring, and kind open and closed questioning
6.1.5	check understanding and use clarification techniques
6.1.6	respond to women's questions and concerns with kindness and compassion
6.1.7	avoid discriminatory behaviour and identify signs of unconscious bias in self and others
6.1.8	use clear language and appropriate resources, making adjustments where appropriate to optimise women's, and their partners' and families', understanding of their own and their newborn infant's health and well-being
6.1.9	recognise the need for, and facilitate access to, translation and interpretation services
6.1.10	recognise and accommodate sensory impairments during all communications
6.2	demonstrate the ability to use evidence-based approaches to build relationships with women, newborn infants, partners and families that respect and enable the woman's needs, views, preferences, and decisions
6.2.1	build and maintain trusting, kind, and respectful professional relationships
6.2.2	convey respect, compassion and sensitivity when supporting women, their partners and families who are emotionally vulnerable and/or distressed
6.2.3	demonstrate the ability to conduct sensitive, individualised conversations that are informed by current evidence on public health promotion strategies
6.2.4	demonstrate effective communication to initiate sensitive, compassionate, woman-centred conversations with pregnant women and new mothers around infant feeding and relationship building
6.2.5	engage effectively in difficult conversations, including conversations about sensitive issues related to ethical dilemmas and breaking bad news, and sexuality, pregnancy, childbirth and the newborn infant
6.2.6	demonstrate the ability to explore with women their attitudes, beliefs and preferences related to childbirth, infant feeding, and parenting, taking into account differing cultural contexts and traditions

6.1.11	support and manage the use of personal communication aids	6.2.7	provide effective and timely communication with women who experience complications and additional care needs, and their partners and families. This includes support, accurate information and updates on changes whilst continuing to listen and respond to their concerns, views, preferences, and decisions
6.1.12	identify the need for alternative communication techniques, and access services to support these		
6.1.13	communicate effectively with interdisciplinary and multiagency teams and colleagues in all settings to support the woman's needs, views, preferences, and decisions		
6.1.14	maintain effective and kind communication techniques with women, partners and families in challenging and emergency situations	6.2.8	communicate complex information regarding a woman's care needs in a clear, concise manner to interdisciplinary and multiagency colleagues and teams
6.1.15	maintain effective communication techniques with interdisciplinary and multiagency teams and colleagues in challenging and emergency situations	6.2.9	consult with, seek help from, and refer to other health and social care professionals both in routine and emergency situations
		6.2.10	demonstrate skills of effective challenge, de-escalation and remaining calm, considering and taking account of the views and decisions made by others

Source: www.nmc.org.uk/

learning disabilities is unknown, Mencap (2022) estimate it to be approximately 2.16 per cent of adults.

Under the Equality Act 2010, people have a legal right to expect services to make changes to remove barriers to accessing healthcare (CQC, 2022). Barriers can be the physical environment, other people's attitudes or information not presented in an understandable way. CQC (2022) found that people with learning disabilities found it difficult to access healthcare because reasonable adjustments had not been made, suggesting reasonable adjustments that support access to services generally should include:

- Familiarisation visits.
- Tailored appointments.
- Adaptation to the physical environment and reduced waiting times.

Continuity of care can also improve engagement with accessing care and support. Taking time to listen and be responsive is key to understanding individual's challenges to support them in their choice of infant feeding. Some people carry a hospital passport (Mencap, 2022) which provides information about the person, likes and dislikes, communication needs and any health conditions or medications. Advocates can help the voice of a parent be heard, help develop relationships and raise awareness of any specific needs. Specialist parenting programmes have also been shown to improve outcomes for parents with learning disabilities.

Mothers with learning disabilities are less likely to breastfeed. Johnson *et al.* (2021) conducted a scoping review to understand how women with learning disabilities can be supported to make infant feeding decisions. Whilst there was a lack of evidence, they did confirm women with learning disabilities need tailored support and accessible resources such as easily read visual images. However, despite being a legal requirement, Homeyard and Patelarou (2018) found fewer than 17 per cent of NHS Trusts in England had accessible antenatal information about breastfeeding and fewer than 50 per cent of midwives routinely offered extra time or follow visits for women with learning disabilities.

Accessible information should be provided in a variety of formats to meet the individuals needs such as:

- Easy read.
- Graphic, animation, DVD or/video clip through accessible websites.
- Large print.
- Face to face meetings (continuity of care when possible).

Discussion of all resources provided is important to ensure they are understood correctly and to avoid vague language and terms that could be misinterpreted.

Autism

Not all people with autism have a diagnosis. People with autism have different ways of communicating and may find it difficult to read social cues and body language. They may take language literally, so it is important to use clear, unambiguous language and phrases and to be patient if questions are repeated. Some people with autism find eye contact uncomfortable, so do not assume they are ignoring you. Some may find physical contact challenging and be misinterpreted as a feeding aversion. It may also make skin-to-skin contact difficult. They may interpret touch as pain or have less sensation of pain, not realising damage is being done to the nipples (BFN, 2014). When asking someone with autism a question, be specific and avoid broad, vague questions as they may be cause anxiety. Environment is important as some people with autism have sensitivity to noise and this may make concentration difficult. They may also like to keep to routines, which may appear to conflict with responsive feeding. The Breastfeeding Network suggest regular checking that communication is clear both ways, and finding strategies for will makes a definite difference to an autistic person's breastfeeding journey.

Hearing impairment

It is imperative that you face a mother with hearing impairment so she can see your mouth. Do not shout but instead speak slowly and clearly, avoiding long and complex sentences. Make sure you have their attention before starting to talk and minimise any distractions or noise that could interfere with hearing aids. Visual aids can support communication such as pictures or white boards. Requesting support from a sign language interpreter may be required.

Further information and detail about the conversations for pregnancy and the postnatal period can be found at Guidance for antenatal and postnatal conversations – BBFI (unicef.org.uk).

Trauma-informed practise

It is important to recognise when someone is affected by trauma and understand the impact. Trauma can refer to a wide range of events that have happened throughout life, such as adverse childhood experiences and abuse in adulthood that are emotionally or physically harmful. Trauma can be understood in terms of the three Es (https://transformingpsychologicaltrauma.scot/resources/understanding-trauma).

- The event.
- How it is experienced.
- Its effects.

'Psychological trauma' refers to the impact on an individual rather than the event itself. Women's response to trauma can vary during the perinatal period and is often the first time they have disclosed it. Some may have experienced a single traumatic event or repeated events over time. Some groups of people at greater risk of experiencing trauma include people living in poverty or insecure housing, refugees and those seeking asylum; Black, Asian and minority ethnic groups; and people who have been trafficked, are homeless, in prison or living with physical or psychological issues and including substance use (Law *et al.*, 2021).

Providing 'trauma-informed' care is underpinned by:

- **R**ealising how common the experience of trauma and adversity is.
- **R**ecognising the different ways that trauma can affect people.
- **R**esponding by taking account of the ways people can be affected by trauma to be able to support recovery.

- Opportunities to resist re-traumatisation and offer a greater sense of choice and control, empowerment, collaboration and safety with everyone that you have contact with.
- Recognising the central importance of relationships.

Eagen-Torkko *et al.* (2017) identified that women with a history of childhood maltreatment and post-traumatic stress disorder are half as likely to breastfeed at six weeks postpartum. Channell Doig *et al.* (2020) conducted a review of 275 articles on breastfeeding and childhood maltreatment to explore how women's experiences affected breastfeeding outcomes. They found that childhood maltreatment was associated with shorter durations of breastfeeding; however, individual experiences of breastfeeding varied from feeling empowered to traumatising. Kendall-Tackett (2017) suggests that if trauma is recent or ongoing, it can activate the stress or inflammation system and can suppress both oxytocin and prolactin. As one in four women disclose having experienced trauma in their lifetimes, using trauma-informed approaches to care may prevent re-traumatisation and support breastfeeding. It should be universal in perinatal care as women may chose not to disclose their experiences.

These key principles of trauma-informed practice (SG, 2021) are from the Trauma-Informed Practice: A Toolkit for Scotland:

1. **Safety:** Efforts are made by an organisation to ensure the physical and emotional safety of clients and staff. This includes reasonable freedom from threat or harm and attempts to prevent further re-traumatisation.
2. **Trustworthiness:** Transparency exists in an organisation's policies and procedures, with the objective of building trust among staff, clients and the wider community.
3. **Choice:** Clients and staff have meaningful choice and a voice in the decision-making process of the organisation and its services.
4. **Collaboration:** The organisation recognises the value of staff and clients' experience in overcoming challenges and improving the system as a whole. This is often operationalised through the formal or informal use of peer support and mutual self-help.
5. **Empowerment:** Efforts are made by the organisation to share power and give clients and staff a strong voice in decision-making, at both individual and organisational levels.

Individuals who have experienced trauma respond to breastfeeding in different ways; for example, if they have experienced sexual abuse, they may fear touching or feeding their babies in case they hurst or harm their babies. It is important to give them time to vocalise their fears and to be aware that new experiences could trigger new reactions.

Law *et al.* (2021) propose four principles of trauma-informed care for the perinatal period:

- Compassion and recognition.
- Communication and collaboration.

- Consistency and continuity.
- Recognising diversity and facilitating recovery.

Further detail can be found at www.england.nhs.uk/wp-content/uploads/2021/02/BBS-TIC-V8.pdf.

> How do your organisation's policies and procedures include a focus on trauma?
> How does your organisation ensure all staff receive basic training on trauma and
> its impact?

Learning about breastfeeding

As discussed in Chapter 1, the lack of knowledge and skills of healthcare professionals is a contributing factor for poor breastfeeding rates. Renfrew *et al.* (2005, 2012), Victora *et al.* (2016), Rollins *et al.* (2016), Gavine *et al.* (2016) and NICE (2021a) recommended that healthcare professionals should be educated using the BFI standards as a minimum. So how do healthcare professionals learn about breastfeeding, and how do they develop a repertoire of skills and knowledge to promote, support and protect breastfeeding?

Breastfeeding knowledge and skills can be influenced by:

- Research.
- Clinical experience.
- Trial and error.
- Habitual practice ('the way things are done around here').
- Personal experience, beliefs, values and attitudes.
- Organisational issues.

Each of these factors is an important component in learning about breastfeeding and decision-making in practice but in isolation can lead to conflicting advice and inappropriate care. There are many theories of adult learning. Fawcett *et al.* (2001) support a holistic approach to learning but also caution against exclusive emphasis on one method of acquiring knowledge and recommend an approach such as Carper's (1978) and White's (1995) to facilitate different ways of viewing and interpreting evidence to put into practice.

Carper (1978, p. 13) believed that to teach and learn about nursing successfully, it was necessary to understand the 'patterns, forms and structure' of the body of knowledge that informs clinical practice. She described four fundamental patterns of knowing, which when used together would ensure nurses and midwives were equipped to provide appropriate, acceptable and holistic care for their clients. She emphasised that the components were interrelated and therefore each was dependent on the others.

- *Empirics, the science of nursing*: a systematic method of enquiry looking at care in an objective way; evidence-based practice. Carper (1978) believed that this was the first fundamental pattern of knowing.

- *Aesthetics, the art of nursing*: This is often misinterpreted as describing the psychomotor skills of practice. Instead, it refers to knowing that is subjective and unique, including creative approaches to care that are not always based on empirical evidence; it is perceiving the client as a whole and responding to their individual needs.
- *The component of personal knowledge*: This is sometimes confused with factual knowledge. However, Carper described personal knowledge as the most essential pattern of knowing, while being the most difficult to teach. Personal knowing is also subjective and is about learning to know ourselves and using experience to develop effective interpersonal skills and learning to understand ourselves and how we relate to others.
- *Ethics, moral knowledge*: Decision-making in clinical practice can be difficult because of the unique nature of individual clinical situations. Carper believed that ethical knowing is more than understanding codes and guidelines and suggested that it included knowing what is right and wrong in the provision of care, particularly when making value judgments.

White (1995) added yet another pattern, 'socio-political', which she believed to be fundamental to all the other patterns. This additional pattern moves the focus from the individual relationship and situates it in a wider context, encouraging the nurse to examine professional practice and the politics of service provision. White (1995) related socio-political knowing to cultural identity and suggested that to understand concepts of health, nurses must have a wider knowledge of the social, political and economic influences on service provision. This pattern is crucial to knowing about breastfeeding where patterns of social and cultural influences are evident in breastfeeding rates in the UK.

Reflective practice

Another way practitioners learn is through reflection. Schön (1983) highlighted reflection as a defining characteristic of a profession. Reflection and reflective practice have become ubiquitous terms in nursing and midwifery practice and are associated with deep learning, but the terms are sometimes confused.

Reflective practice links theory to practice by consciously thinking through experiences (Howatson-Jones, 2016, p. 10). Practitioners learn through experience and, through the process of reflection, identify how they feel about the situation in light of current knowledge and are then able to plan for future action. Heath (1998) suggested that when problems are complex, reflection may assist nurses and midwives to develop a reasoned argument for a change in practice. Boud *et al.* (1985) claimed that structured reflection is key to learning from experience and described three stages students go through: preparation, engagement and processing, including reflective activity at each stage.

Schön (1983) divided the process of reflection into two categories: 'reflection-on-action' and 'reflection-in-action'. Reflection-on-action refers to the practice of thinking critically about an event after it has occurred, while reflection-in-action, which is usually only evident in the competent practitioner, occurs while carrying out a procedure or providing care, often unconsciously, but demonstrating that the practitioner is using creative approaches within individual situations.

There are many different models to aid the process of reflection, and it is personal preference as to which is used. Gibbs' (1998) reflective cycle is commonly used by students due to its simple and structured step-by-step approach (Figure 12.2).

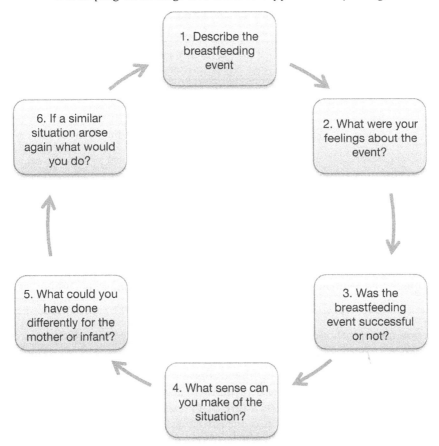

Figure 12.2 Reflecting on a breastfeeding event
Source: adapted from Gibbs (1998).

Another commonly used model for reflection was developed by Johns, who compiled a set of questions based around Carper's (1978) four patterns of knowing (Table 12.2) with the aim of encouraging the practitioner to be reflexive about their practice and adaptable to new situations. In contrast to Carper, Johns (1995) identified aesthetics to be at the root of knowing and that the empirical, personal and ethical knowing all inform the holistic response to a clinical situation. He suggested that to provide individualised care, the nurse must interpret the empirical evidence to suit the clinical situation rather than the other way around. Johns (1995) developed cue questions to aid practitioners to make sense of their experiences and to identify the areas of knowing that are required to provide effective, safe and satisfying care for clients.

The current focus on objective, empirical evidence, in which randomised controlled trials are seen as the gold standard, has led to concerns that nurses and midwives may not be able to respond fully to the complex and diverse nature of clinical situations with which they are faced. Paley *et al.* (2007) conducted a comprehensive literature review to compare nursing's patterns of knowing with those of cognitive science, establishing that scientific knowledge still had priority over other forms of knowledge. However, for care to

Table 12.2 Summary of Johns' model of structured reflection (1995) in relation to Carper's (1978) four patterns of knowing

Carper's four patterns of knowing in nursing	Johns' cue questions for reflection
Empirics	What knowledge did inform or should have informed me?
Aesthetics	What was I trying to achieve?
	Why did I respond as I did?
	What were the consequences for the client? Others? Myself?
	How did the client feel?
	How did I know this?
Personal knowing	How did I feel in this situation?
	What internal factors were influencing me?
Ethics	How did my actions match with my beliefs?
	What factors made me act in incongruent ways?

be meaningful and effective, objective empirical knowledge cannot be exclusive. It cannot provide the answers to all practice questions and needs to be considered alongside other forms of qualitative evidence as well as the other patterns of knowing (White, 1995).

Reflection on parenthood education class using Gibbs' reflective cycle

Description: Describe what happened during the breastfeeding event.
I had been asked to take a local parenthood education class for multiparous women in an area of high unemployment and deprivation to discuss breastfeeding. Breastfeeding rates in this area are low and I was aware that all the women had previously bottle-fed. I wanted to discuss the benefits of breastfeeding without causing any offence.

I explained about the research that has been carried out in relation to the benefits for mother and baby. I did not want anyone to feel guilty about their previous choice of infant feeding and tried to make the session quite lighthearted. Most of the women appeared receptive to the idea that breast was best, but one woman, Mrs B, was very confrontational, insisting that her previous child was healthy and that she and all her family had been bottle fed and turned out all right and that breastfeeding was for middle-class women.

Feelings: What were you thinking or feeling during the event?
Initially, I was very nervous that I would cause offence but felt confident in the information I was supplying. However, when Mrs B became confrontational and unwilling to take my message on board, I felt very self-conscious and uncomfortable. I did not want to embarrass her but had to continue and present the evidence to support breastfeeding and highlight the dangers inherent in bottle feeding.

Evaluation: What went well or not so well in this event?
I had prepared well for the session, using up-to-date evidence-based material to address the outcomes of the session that had been given to me by the person who normally takes the class. I had made a lesson plan and ensured that I kept to time. I felt the session was light hearted while getting the message across to most of the group. I introduced the topic, said what I was going to say, said it and then summed it up at the end. The other women appeared to listen.

However, Mrs B was quite verbally aggressive and unwilling to listen or discuss the issues. My intention had been to provide the group with information that they may not have received before and to get them to think about the possibility of breastfeeding and to support them to address the challenges they may face. Unfortunately, Mrs B was quite disruptive, and I found the session very challenging. I was embarrassed and found it difficult to reply to her statements.

Analysis: What sense can you make out of the situation? Break it down into parts to explore in more detail.

The result of the session was that both Mrs B and I left the session unsatisfied and that Mrs B had not taken in any of the information I had provided. I felt that I had been unable to deal with her confrontational attitude and that it had disrupted the session for the other women. I realise that it was not Mrs B's intention to be disruptive and that she probably felt I was attacking the choices she and her family had previously made.

I have discussed the episode with other clinicians and feel that I should have made the session more interactive, facilitating the discussion rather than just presenting information. For example, I could have done this by using the 'benefits of breastfeeding' poster as a visual aid to start the discussion about the benefits of breastfeeding for both mother and baby to prompt further discussion. I could also have given each woman a locally produced leaflet to take home to discuss with her family.

Conclusion: Now you have looked at it from different angles, is there anything else you could have done or should not have done?

I realise that situations like this will always arise. It is probable that I took the wrong approach and could have presented the evidence in a more user-friendly and interactive way. Maybe the language I used was inappropriate, as was my presentation style, and Mrs B could have misinterpreted it and felt I was being condescending.

Action plan: What would you do differently in a similar situation?

I feel more aware of the need to tailor the session for the client group, and instead of presenting information, I will make the session more interactive. The next time I conduct a session, I will ask someone to attend with me for support and to give me some critical feedback.

Evidence-based practice

'Evidence-based practice' has also become a ubiquitous term in nursing and midwifery practice, but there is often confusion between the terms evidence-based practice, audit and research:

- Research is the systematic search to discover new information.
- Evidence-based practice uses the best available evidence to provide effective care.
- Audit is the process for reviewing care against best practice standards.

Evidence-based care is described as 'doing the right things right' (Gray, 2001) and 'the conscientious, explicit and judicious use of current best evidence in making decisions about the care of individual patients' (Sackett *et al.*, 1996, p. 71). Grove *et al.* identify the elements of evidence-based practice as based on:

- Best research evidence.
- Clinical expertise.
- Patient needs and values.

(Grove *et al.*, 2014)

A variety of evidence can be used when deciding on the most appropriate line of care for mothers who are breastfeeding, but it must be assessed in conjunction with the individual event or situation, which will include psychosocial factors as well as physical ones. Healthcare professionals must be able to evaluate the strength of evidence identifying reliability, validity and generalisability; this is commonly done by rating research in a hierarchy of evidence (Figure 12.3).

The Cochrane Library database contains regularly updated systematic reviews prepared by the Cochrane Collaboration (www.cochrane.org). A systematic review can be described as a literature review of the available studies on a particular subject, which is then analysed and synthesised, resulting in an objective conclusion about the cost-effectiveness and appropriateness of interventions or treatments. If the results are inconclusive, the recommendation for further research may be made (Parahoo, 2014).

The aim of systematic reviews is to remove errors of interpretation and bias. Any misleading information and unsupported opinions are also likely to be removed. However, not all breastfeeding problems are capable of being solved by scientific means, resulting in limited available evidence. Evidence-based practice may offer some solutions and suggest a way forward, but it is not an answer for all the situations that professionals may encounter and therefore can limit the choice for both the expert and the mother, as the professional cannot justify using non-researched practices. This is evident throughout this book, when evidence is limited in support of some areas of practice. Other useful sources of breastfeeding information can be found later in this chapter in the section 'Finding the evidence', and resources specific to breastfeeding can be found at the end of each chapter.

Healthcare professionals must not rely on systematic reviews alone and need to learn critical appraisal skills themselves. All graduate programmes thread research through curricula. This includes how to critically review literature and appraise evidence-based practice. Critical appraisal skills are essentially the skills required to read research papers and make decisions about their reliability, validity and generalisability of evidence.

Clinical guidelines and policies are based on the best available evidence at the time. These can be national guidelines such as those published by NICE or locally developed

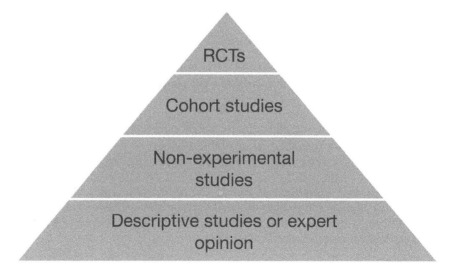

Figure 12.3 The hierarchy of evidence. RCT = randomized controlled trial.

guidance. Clinical guidelines are usually presented as detailed protocols, clinical pathways for groups of patients or algorithms to aid decision-making.

Activity

There are a number of issues you might wish to consider in relation to your place of study or work.

- Do you know how to access online databases and journals?
- Can you search for and find the appropriate literature to answer your questions adequately?
- Do you have the appropriate skills and knowledge to make judgments about the evidence you collect?
- Do you have an Athens account? MyAthens (openathens.net) or equivalent.

If you are having problems with any of these areas, make an appointment with your subject librarian, who will be happy to help you.

Finding the evidence

It is important to know where to look for evidence and to be able to access it. In recent years, there have been a number of online developments in this area for healthcare professionals. Listen next are some useful sites you can access. Remember to use librarians to help you as they have a wealth of information and are happy to help you to improve your ability to search for literature.

The Cochrane Database of Systematic Reviews contains regularly updated systematic reviews prepared by the Cochrane Collaboration: www.cochrane.org.

The National Institute for Health and Clinical Excellence (NICE) is an independent organisation responsible for providing national guidance on promoting good health and preventing and treating ill health: www.nice.org.uk.

Health Education England Knowledge and Library Hub is a gateway to many sources of health information for healthcare professionals: https://library.hee.nhs.uk/resources/nhs-knowledge-and-library-hub.

Health Education and Improvement Wales (HEIW) provides information on policies for Wales. It has a useful publications section for accessing policy documents: heiw.nhs.wales.

NIdirect provides information on Northern Ireland policies. It has a useful publications section for accessing policy documents: www.health-ni.gov.uk.

The Nursing and Midwifery Council (NMC) provides access to publications and policies relevant to nursing and professional practice: www.nmc.org.uk.

The Royal College of Midwifery (RCM) provides access to online journals and has related evidence on professional issues: www.rcm.org.uk.

The Royal College of Nursing (RCN) provides access to online journals and has related evidence on professional issues: www.rcn.org.uk.

The Knowledge Network is the national online library and knowledge service for health and social care in Scotland provided by NHS Education for Scotland: www.knowledge.scot.nhs.uk.

The Scottish Government provides information on policies for Scotland. It has a useful publications section for accessing policy documents: www.gov.scot.

The World Health Organization (WHO) is the directing and coordinating authority for health within the United Nations system. It is responsible for providing leadership on global health matters, shaping the health research agenda, setting norms and standards, articulating evidence-based policy options, providing technical support to countries and monitoring and assessing health trends: www.who.int.

Concluding comments

Communication skills are key to supporting mothers with breastfeeding to provide them with clear, accurate information that they can understand and use to help them continue breastfeeding for as long as they would like to. Doing this will empower mothers to make informed choices on the most appropriate care for them, their infants and their families. However, it must be remembered that, as there are numerous sources of information today, particularly from the internet, care must be taken to ensure that information is from reputable sources.

Reflective questions

1 Using your own choice of reflective model, reflect on a recent episode of care when supporting a mother with breastfeeding when you can identify the use of Carper's four patterns of learning. Highlight where you obtained the evidence to support your practice and where it fits into the hierarchy of evidence.
2 Keep a reflective journal to provide evidence of your learning for your personal portfolio. This will enable you to organise your thoughts and encourage self-awareness and exploration of your actions or omissions in providing care for breastfeeding mothers.

Further reading

- National Trauma Training Programme: https://transformingpsychologicaltrauma. scot/.
- A good practice guide to support implementation of trauma-informed care in the perinatal period: www.england.nhs.uk/wp-content/uploads/2021/02/BBS-TIC-V8. pdf.
- CHANGE – Learning Disability Rights Charity – Easy Read (changepeople.org) have a range of easy read Parenting Collection resources including 'My Choice, My Pregnancy', 'You and Your Baby, 0–1'.
- Best Beginnings. (2021). Parents with learning disabilities www.bestbeginnings. org.uk/parents-with-learning-disabilities.
- Easy Read: All about breastfeeding All about breastfeeding For new mothers in North Wales (nhs.wales).

Appendix 1

UNICEF UK Baby Friendly Initiative
University Standards (2019a)

Theme 1: Understand breastfeeding

1 Have sufficient knowledge of anatomy of the breast and physiology of lactation to enable them to support mothers to successfully establish and maintain breastfeeding.
2 Understand the importance of human milk and breastfeeding to the health and wellbeing outcomes of mothers, babies and the wider family.

Topics to include:

- Anatomy of the breast and changes in pregnancy.
- Physiology of lactation and hormonal influences on both milk production and instinctive mothering behaviour.
- The role of the Feedback Inhibitor of Lactation (FIL).
- Fetal glucose homeostasis and counter-regulation.
- Breastfeeding and public health; for the mother and baby, as well as the societal, environmental and economic impact.
- The role that breastfeeding and human milk play in improving the health and wellbeing outcomes of babies, their mothers and the wider family.
- Constituents of colostrum and breastmilk, including protective and developmental factors Constituent differences between human milk and infant formula.
- Epigenetics and the microbiome related to infant feeding and very early child development.
- Applying theory to practice; implications for current midwifery and health visiting practice.

Theme 2: Support infant feeding

3 Have an understanding of infant feeding culture within the UK and the various influences and constraints which impact on women's infant feeding decisions.
4 Be able to apply their knowledge and understanding of the physiology of lactation to support women to get breastfeeding off to a good start.
5 Be able to apply their knowledge of physiology and the principle of reciprocity to support mothers to keep their babies close and respond to their cues for feeding, love and comfort.
6 Have the knowledge and skills to support mothers and babies to maximise breastmilk and breastfeeding, to continue to breastfeed for as long as they wish and to introduce solid foods at an appropriate time.

7 Be able to support parents who formula feed to do so responsively and as safely as possible.
8 Understand the importance of the WHO International Code of Marketing of Breast-milk Substitutes and subsequent WHA resolutions (the Code) and how it impacts on practice.

Topics to include:

- Overview of infant feeding culture in the UK and what has influenced changing breast-feeding rates in the UK and worldwide.
- Importance of skin-to-skin contact to support a good start to breastfeeding and mother-ing (for all mothers irrespective of feeding type) and how to facilitate this within practice.
- Responsive breastfeeding and how mothers and babies develop a reciprocal relation-ship when they remain close (to include feeding and comfort cues).
- How a baby breastfeeds – understanding principles and mechanisms of attachment and positioning for effective feeding.
- How to support mothers and babies as they 'learn' to breastfeed including an under-standing of instinctive behaviour, e.g. laid back breastfeeding.
- Recognising effective breastfeeding; assessing milk production and milk transfer, as-sessing a breastfeed in practice.
- Supporting breastfeeding mothers to maximise the amount of breastmilk their baby receives.
- Responsive bottle feeding, including how to hold a baby during a bottle feed and how to pace the feeds.
- Support parents who are bottle feeding to minimise the risks, to make up feeds safely and understand how to sterilise equipment.
- For mothers who are formula feeding, how and where to access independent informa-tion on infant formula.
- Appropriate introduction of other foods including developmental readiness, ways to feed and achieving a balanced diet.
- Practical skills reviews.
- Evidenced-based interventions that promote, support and protect breastfeeding – including the WHO/UNICEF Baby Friendly Initiative.
- The WHO International Code of Marketing of Breastmilk Substitutes and subsequent resolutions: rationale, history and impact on practice.

Theme 3: Support close and loving relationships

9 Develop an understanding of the importance of secure mother-infant attachment and the impact this has on their health and emotional wellbeing.
10 Be able to apply their knowledge of attachment theory to promote and encourage close and loving relationships between babies, their mothers and families, irrespective of their feeding method.

Topics to include:

- Overview of infant brain development and the importance of love and nurture to en-sure optimal outcomes.

- Overview of attachment theories and how this applies to practice.
- Supporting parents through pregnancy, birth and beyond to develop close and loving relationships with their baby.

Theme 4: Manage the challenges

11 Be able to apply their knowledge of the physiology of lactation and infant feeding to support effective management of challenges which may arise at any time during breastfeeding.
12 Have an understanding of the special circumstances which can affect lactation and breastfeeding (e.g. when mother and baby are separated, including preterm and sick infants) and be able to support mothers to overcome the challenges.
13 Draw on their knowledge and understanding of the wider social, cultural and political influences which undermine breastfeeding, to promote, support and protect breast-feeding within their sphere of practice.

Topics to include:

- Manage common breastfeeding challenges for both mother and baby e.g. sore nipples, engorgement, mastitis, thrush, insufficient milk supply, hypoglycaemia, jaundice etc., including appropriate referral.
- Expression of breastmilk to include hand and pump expression technique.
- Initiating and sustaining lactation when mother and baby are separated including sick and preterm infants.
- Supporting parents to stay with and care for their baby in transitional and neonatal care.
- Maximising human milk feeding and breastfeeding where breastfeeding may be compromised.
- Supporting breastfeeding where there are maternal health issues.
- Role of specialist infant feeding support, peer support groups and the voluntary organisations.
- Situations when breastfeeding is not recommended, use of donor human milk.
- Normalising breastfeeding: protecting, promoting and supporting breastfeeding; exploring the politics of breastfeeding that impact on practice and care of women.

Theme 5: Promote positive communication

14 Have an understanding of the principles of effective communication and current thinking around public health promotion strategies and approaches.
15 Be able to apply their knowledge of effective communication to initiate sensitive, com-passionate, mother-centred conversations with pregnant women and new mothers.
16 Have the knowledge and skills to access the evidence-based information that under-pins infant feeding practice and know how to keep up-to-date (e.g. e-alerts, research summaries).

Topics to include:

- Debrief of students' personal infant feeding stories.
- Effective communication skills; theory and practice.

- Importance of an authentic presence, listening and reflecting back for effective communication.
- Importance of compassion, sensitivity and kindness Public health theory and practice; supporting women to make informed decisions, creating an environment where behaviour change is possible.
- Mother-centred care; theory and practice.
- Skills development to support midwives and health visitors to facilitate conversations with pregnant women, new mothers and families.
- Skills to support families where English is not the first language.
- Skills required for providing telephone support.
- Working with others in a multidisciplinary environment to support infant feeding.
- Sensitive communication of safer sleep messages.

Appendix 2

Nursing and Midwifery Council *Standards for Proficiency for Midwives* (2019)

NMC Standards of proficiency for midwives (2019)

Key themes

- evidence-based care and the importance of staying up-to-date with current knowledge.
- the physical, psychological, social, cultural, and spiritual safety of women and newborn infants.
- communication and relationship building, working in partnership with women.
- enabling and advocating for the human rights of women and children.
- enabling and advocating for the views, preferences, and decisions of women, partners and families.
- working across the whole continuum of care and in all settings, and understanding the woman's and newborn infant's whole maternity journey.
- providing continuity of care and carer.
- optimising the normal processes of reproduction and early life.
- ensuring that women, partners and families have all the information needed to fully inform their decisions.
- the importance of physical, psychological, social, cultural, and spiritual factors.
- anticipating, preventing, and responding to complications and additional care needs.
- public health, health promotion, and health protection.
- understanding and working to mitigate health and social inequalities.
- interdisciplinary and multiagency working.
- **protecting, promoting and supporting breastfeeding.**
- the impact of pregnancy, labour and birth, postpartum, infant feeding, and the early weeks of life on longer-term health and well-being.
- taking personal responsibility for ongoing learning and development.

Domain 3: universal care for all women and newborn infants

A.   *The midwife's role in public health, health promotion and health protection*

3.6   understand the importance of human milk and breastfeeding to public health and well-being, and demonstrate how to protect, promote and enable breastfeeding with the woman, her partner and family.

Domain 4: additional care for women and newborn infants with complication

A.   *The midwife's role in first line assessment and management of complications and additional care needs*

4.5   demonstrate knowledge, understanding, and the ability to recognise complications and additional care needs of the woman and/or newborn infant, in regard to infant feeding and the implications of feeding for very early child development.

Domain 6: the midwife as a skilled practitioner

Assessment, screening, planning, care and support across the continuum: shared skills for Domains 3 and 4.

6.46   assess, promote, and encourage the development of the mother-newborn infant relationship, and opportunities for attachment, contact, interaction, and relationship building between the woman, newborn infant, partner and family.

6.47   enable immediate, uninterrupted, and ongoing safe skin-to-skin contact between the mother and the newborn infant, and positive time for the partner and family to be with the newborn infant and each other, preventing unnecessary interruptions.

6.48   observe, assess, and promote the woman's, and partner's (as appropriate), immediate response to the newborn infant, and their ability to keep the newborn infant close and be responsive to the newborn infant's cues for love, comfort and feeding (reciprocity).

Appendix 3

UNICEF UK BFI *Neonatal Standards* (2022)

Stage 1: building a firm foundation 1

1 Have written policies and guidelines to support the standards.
2 Plan and education programme what will allow staff to implement the standards according to their role.
3 Have processes for implementing, auditing and evaluating the standards.
4 Ensure that there is no promotion of breastmilk substitutes, bottles, teats or dummies in any part of the facility or by any of the staff.

Stage 2: an educated workforce

1 Educate staff to implement the standards according to their role and the service provided.

Stage 3: parents' experiences of neonatal units

1 **Support parents to have a close and loving relationship with their baby.**

   1) Parents understand why close and loving relationships are important now and in the long term.
   2) In the absence of parents, baby's needs for comfort and emotional support are met by an individual selected by the parents or by a staff member.
   3) Parents and staff are enabled to recognise baby's behavioural cues and tolerance for stimulus and parents are supported to build close relationships via touch, talking, comforting, etc. as appropriate.
   4) Prolonged, frequent skin-to-skin contact is encouraged for all babies. Skin contact is prevented only for acceptable clinical reasons and not because of a lack of staff training or resources.
   5) Parents and staff who are bottle feeding are supported to do this responsively, recognising the baby's cues and need for comfort and closeness during feeding.

2 **Enable babies to receive breastmilk and to breastfeed when possible.**

   1) A discussion with parents takes place about the value of breastmilk as early as possible.
   2) Mother's own breastmilk is always the first choice of feed (except for a small number of acceptable clinical indications, for example HIV infection or a mother undergoing chemotherapy).

3) Mothers are enabled to express milk as soon as possible, ideally within the first two hours.
4) Breastmilk is used for mouth care and tempting the baby to feed.
5) Mothers learn how to express effectively by hand and pump (as appropriate to individual need) and learn how to store milk.
6) Mothers are supported to express frequently to optimise supply, especially in first 2–3 weeks.
7) Mothers have access to adequate and effective expressing equipment to use on the unit and at home.
8) A formal review of expressing takes place a minimum of four times in the first two weeks and there is access to further help with expressing if milk supplies are inadequate or less than 750 mls by day 10.
9) Expressing is frequently checked on an informal basis after the first two weeks.
10) The unit has an environment conducive to expressing.
11) Skin contact is used to induce instinctive feeding behaviours.
12) Mothers can be close to their baby in order to respond to feeding cues.
13) Support with positioning and attachment and recognising effective feeding.
14) Additional support is provided to help with expressing and feeding challenges when needed, including specialist help when required.
15) Mothers are prepared for going home.
16) Information about how to access support with feeding in the community.
17) There is no advertising for breastmilk substitutes, bottles, teats or dummies.

3 **Value parents as partners in care.**

1) There is a policy of 24 hour access; staff routines and practices do not interfere with this.
2) Measures are taken to ensure that practical difficulties do not prevent parents being with their baby.
3) Parents are welcomed on the unit and treated with dignity, respect and equality.
4) Parents are respected as primarily responsible for their child. Their opinion is sought and they are involved in decision making.
5) Parents are enabled to carry out as much of the care as possible.
6) Parents are encouraged to comfort and support their baby during procedures.

Full guidance is available at www.unicef.org.uk/babyfriendly/

Appendix 4

Answers to quizzes and scenarios

Chapter 3

True or false quiz

1	False	The size of the breast is determined by the amount of fatty tissue. This does not predict milk storage capacity.
2	True	Storage capacity is variable, but over a 24-hour period, all lactating mothers produce approximately average 750–800 ml/24 hours. Those with lower storage capacity feed more frequently than their counterparts.
3	True	Ramsay claimed the lactiferous ducts branch off within the areola and found no evidence of lactiferous sinuses.
4	False	Geddes claims mothers can have multiple milk ejections during a feed ranging from 0–9.
5	False	Water makes up about 80 per cent of milk volume, and therefore infants do not need supplements. Supplements interfere with milk production.
6	True	Colostrum has a purgative effect on the bowel and helps clear meconium.
7	True	As the feed progresses, the fat level gradually increases.
8	False	Secretory immunoglobulin A (sIgA), entero- and broncho-mammary pathways, white blood cells and antibodies from previous maternal infections cannot be replicated in formula milk.
9	True	Prolactin is inhibited until the delivery of the placenta and membranes (complete), resulting in decreased levels of progesterone, oestrogen, HPL and PIF.
10	False	A build-up of FIL will decrease milk production, and therefore the breasts should be emptied on a regular basis.

Chapter 4

Quiz

1 Sustainable position; head and neck in a straight line; allow infant to move her or his head freely; hold the infant close; nose to nipple; lead with the chin.
2 The underarm position.
3 Wide mouth; chin indents the breast; lower lip curled out; full cheeks; hear swallowing; see milk at the mouth; more areola at top than bottom.
4 Cheeks drawn in; both lips flanged; long or short feeds with an unsettled infant; explosive, watery, frothy stool; failure to thrive; nipple trauma; breast refusal.
5 At the end of the feed.

6 A minimum of two breastfeeding assessments be carried out in the first week to ensure the infant is feeding well- urine and stool, position; attachment and sucking pattern; breasts and nipples. This should be followed by a plan of care.
7 Assess urine and stools and weight.
8 At least eight times, including nighttime when prolactin levels are high.
9 Wash hands and prepare storage equipment; comfortable position, massage breasts; feel around areola for difference in consistency; place thumb and first two fingers in a 'C' shape and gently compress at 6 and 12 o'clock about 2–3 cm above the nipple; compress and release. As milk ejection ceases move to another position.
10 Increases prolactin levels and saves time.

Chapter 5

Scenario 1

- It is vital that Jane is aware of the many benefits offered by skin-to-skin contact for any age of infant. It will reduce crying in the baby and stabilise vital signs and provide access to the breast.
- You could suggest co-bathing; this may well be very useful for Jane in settling the baby and having some relaxation in a bath, too.
- Consider safe bed-sharing (Lullaby Trust) – provide Jane with the evidence relating to breastfeeding and SIDS, and if she makes the informed choice to take her baby into bed with her, explain the ways she can reduce the risk of accidents and overheating.

Scenario 2

- Obviously, Sharmila has been through a huge ordeal and is exhausted; she needs lots of positive feedback on how well she has done.
- A ask her to feed her baby again, giving her full support and encouragement. Observe a breastfeed for all the signs of effective positioning and attachment, as there may be a simple problem that has led to the situation of the baby feeding frequently.
- Is there family there who can cuddle the baby? If not, settle the baby beside her following the feed.
- Explain you wouldn't recommend a dummy until feeding was established because she will be unable to learn her baby's feeding cues and may reduce her milk production if the baby reduces the number of feeds.
- Ensure that Sharmila has effective analgesia and that her vital signs are all within normal limits.
- Maybe there are a lot of visitors, and this may need to be monitored to ensure that Sharmila is given time to recover.

Quiz

1 Sedated from maternal drugs in labour; undiagnosed illness; too hot or cold; feeding cues are missed; separated from mother.
2 Encourages breastfeeding; reduces crying; regulates temperature, respiratory rate and heart rate; promotes bonding.
3 Do not co-sleep on the sofa or bring the infant into bed if you smoke, have taken alcohol or drugs, you or the infant are ill (preterm infants) or you are extremely tired.

Firm mattress; ensure infant cannot be trapped between you and the wall or fall out of bed; do not overdress the infant or leave him or her alone in bed; loose covers that do not go over the head; room temperature 16–18°C. No pets, or other children in the bed with the baby.

4 Helps recognise feeding cues; facilitates unrestricted feeds; improves maternal confidence.

5 Reduces conflicting advice; ensures practice is consistent with WHO Code and UNICEF UK BFI standards; commitment from managers to implement good practice.

6 Posters, leaflets, verbal information.

7 To avoid using a dummy while establishing breastfeeding, particularly within the first month, because it may cause nipple confusion, reduce the number of feeds and decrease milk supply, and the mother is unable to recognise feeding cues. It is also a potential portal for thrush and can lead to tooth decay and recurrent ear infections.

8 Responsive feeding is the reciprocal relationship between mother and infant. The mother learns and responds to the infant's cues to enhance growth, development and emotional attachment.

9 Supplementary feeds lead to reduced suckling and breast stimulation, reduced prolactin production, increased FIL and a decrease in milk supply.

10 Infant cues: sucking movements and noises, licking lips, head movements from side to side, rapid eye movement, restlessness. Crying is a late sign.

Chapter 6

Scenario 1

Determine the cause of the problem by taking a lactation history, examine Daisy's breasts and the infant's mouth for signs of any anomalies and observe a complete breastfeed. Remind her to let the infant come off the breast and how to break the vacuum first if attachment is incorrect. Teach her the principles of position and attachment again and explain that to maintain the milk supply, she also needs to continue to breastfeed or express from the affected side. Recommend different positions that she may find more comfortable.

Scenario 2

Remind Alison of the benefits of breastfeeding for herself and Eve. Take a lactation history and find out if she has support from family and friends to continue breastfeeding. Ask her for a history of the feeding pattern and if anything has changed, such as introducing a dummy or giving supplementary feeds. Determine if there is effective milk transfer by observing a breastfeed and assessing Eve's nappies and weight. Teach Alison the principles of position and attachment again and how to assess milk transfer. Recommend she tries skin-to-skin contact and ensure that Eve is getting a full feed, receiving the fattier milk at the end of the feed.

Scenario 3

Determine the cause of the problem by taking a lactation history and observing a breastfeed. Inform Bridget that to maintain her milk supply, she must breastfeed regularly from both sides and avoid anything that applies pressure on the breast (e.g. tight bra). If she is unable to feed from the affected side, then she should express regularly. Advise her on changing position to aid drainage of the breast. Remind her about the principles of effective position and attachment and how to avoid blocked ducts. Recommend fluids and rest and advise her that she can take analgesia (ibuprofen and paracetamol). If the problem does not improve in 12–14 hours or there is a fissure, she may need antibiotics. If severe or recurrent, a sample for culture should be taken.

Chapter 7

Scenario 1

- Assess a breastfeed (see Chapter 6). Stacey has several risk factors: caesarean section, diabetes, postpartum haemorrhage, large blood loss, blood transfusion.
- Harry had a few risk factors for weight loss: limited skin-to-skin initially, reluctant to feed and he had a few cup feeds.
- Observe a complete breastfeed for position and attachment and milk transfer.
- Discuss responsive feeding, position and attachment and how to recognise feeding cues. Recommend that she avoid using teats and dummies.
- See Chapter 8 for managing weight loss, as this is a 10 per cent loss.
- Encourage skin-to-skin contact.
- Stacey should regularly feed Harry and frequently express to improve her supply of milk; this should include at least once at night.
- Plan to weigh regularly and observe milk transfer.

Scenario 2

COVID-19 vaccination remains the best way to protect both mother and baby from COVID-19, and there is good evidence showing no adverse effects on babies following maternal vaccination. Vaccination is still recommended whilst breastfeeding.

Chapter 8

Scenario 1

- Encourage skin-to-skin and rooming-in so Carol can pick up infant feeding cues.
- Encourage regular breastfeeds, at no more than three-hourly intervals, to increase bowel motility, clear meconium and reduce the reabsorption of unconjugated bilirubin. Advise Carol to wake Amy for feeds.
- Observe and assess breastfeeds to ensure adequate milk transfer.
- If the infant has difficulty feeding, weight loss is more than 7 per cent of the birth weight or there are signs of dehydration, Carol should be encouraged to express breastmilk following the feed and give this as a supplement or 'top-up' rather than formula and give it by cup rather than bottle.

Scenario 2

- Take a full breastfeeding history to discover if there is a feeding problem. Observe positioning and attachment to see if there may be a problem, for example with tongue-tie.
- Is there any history of thrush, etc.?

- Has home life changed? Is Lizzie under stress? What other children does she have? Does she have a supportive family? What is her physical health like?
- Recommend skin-to-skin contact.
- Use a breast pump to increase lactation so she can supplement the breastfeed and increase her milk supply and gradually reduce amounts of formula.
- Assess Frank's nappies; are they wet, dirty? What colour is the stool?
- It may be useful to mention fenugreek and other remedies (if taking other medication, discuss with the GP).
- Close follow-up and reweighing over the next two weeks are very important.
- Use of a cup instead of a teat to supplement as necessary.

Chapter 10

Scenario

- Compliment Khushi on how well she has done with her exclusive breastfeeding and comment on how healthy the baby looks and that she is gaining weight beautifully.
- Advise Khushi to continue exclusive breastfeeding for six months rather than introducing solids at this time.
- Be understanding about the well-meaning relatives who have offered this advice but remind Khushi about the benefits of longer term breastfeeding and the problems that introducing solid food will have on her milk supply and the risk of triggering allergies and increasing the risk of childhood diabetes and obesity.
- Remind Khushi about the signs of being ready to wean, for example, reaching out to grab things, putting things to her mouth and so on. If the baby is not demonstrating these traits and doesn't like the mashed food, it may reassure Khushi that she is not ready to be weaned.

Glossary

Alveoli   Glands within the breast that produce milk. Tiny sacs that look like a bunch of grapes.

Aminoacidopathy   Any inborn error of amino acid metabolism that results in an accumulation of one or more amino acids in the blood or excess excretion in the urine, or both.

Apoptosis   When the secretory epithelial cells die and are reabsorbed.

Autocrine response   When a cell secretes a hormone or chemical that acts on itself.

Complementary feeding   The introduction of foods and drinks after six months of age. These foods are in addition to adequate intake of breastmilk.

Erythema   Redness of the skin.

Exclusive breastfeeding   When an infant receives only breastmilk from its mother or expressed or donor breastmilk. No other liquids or solids, except vitamins or medicines, are given.

Fissure   Crack or tear in the skin.

Galactopoesis   Maintenance of lactation once it has been established.

Glucogenesis   Breakdown of glycogen to form glucose.

Hepatosplenomegaly   Enlargement of the liver and spleen.

Ketogenesis   Production of ketone bodies resulting from fatty acid breakdown.

Lactocyte   Milk-producing cell.

Lactogenesis   The initiation of milk production.

Let-down reflex   Involuntary reflex that causes milk ejection.

Lipolysis   The breakdown of fat into glycerol and fatty acids as a source of energy.

Myoepithelial cells   Smooth muscle around the alveoli that contracts to stimulate milk ejection.

Neuroendocrine response   Interaction between nervous system and endocrine system.

Oedema   Accumulation of extracellular fluid.

Oxytocin   Pituitary hormone that stimulates contraction of the myoepithelial cells around the alveoli to stimulate milk ejection.

Prolactin   Pituitary hormone that stimulates and maintains milk production.

Prolactin inhibiting factor   Hypothalamic substance that inhibits the synthesis and release of prolactin.

Responsive feeding   A two-way relationship between a mother and her baby. The mother responds when her baby shows feeding cues.

Sucking   Action of drawing the breast into the mouth to create a vacuum.

Suckling   Combined characteristics of feeding at the breast, including sucking, swallowing and breathing.

Supplementary feeding Feeds given to a baby younger than six months old to supplement the intake of breastmilk when it is insufficient.

Tongue-tie Abnormal shortness or thickness of the frenulum that results in restricted tongue movement or anchorage to the base of the mouth.

References

Abedi, P., Jahanfar, S., Namvar, F., *et al.* (2016) Breastfeeding or nipple stimulation for reducing postpartum haemorrhage in the third stage of labour, *Cochrane Database of Systematic Reviews*. Available online at https://doi.org/10.1002/14651858.CD010845.pub2 (accessed 18 January 2023)

Adamson, J. (2004) Implementing informed choice on infant feeding, British Journal of Midwifery, 12(9): 586–690

Adsit, J. and Hewlings, S. (2022) Impact of bariatric surgery on breastfeeding: A systematic review, *Surgery for Obesity and Related Diseases*, 18(1): 117–122

The All-Party Parliamentary Group on Infant Feeding & Inequalities (APPG) (2018) *Inquiry into the Cost of Infant Formula in the United Kingdom.* Available online at www.infantfeedingappg.uk/ (accessed 1 October 2022)

Alm, B., Wennergren, G., Möllberg, H., *et al.* (2015) Breastfeeding and dummy use have a protective effect on sudden infant death syndrome, *Acta Paediatrica*, 105(1): 31–38

Almutairi, W. (2021) Review literature review: Physiological management for preventing postpartum hemorrhage, *Healthcare*, 9(658): 1–11

Almutairi, W., Ludington, S., Quinn Griffin, M., *et al.* (2020) The role of skin-to skin contact and breastfeeding on atonic postpartum hemorrhage, *Nursing Reports*, *11*: 1–11

Aloysius, A. and Lozano, S. (2007) Provision of nipple shields to preterm infants on a neonatal unit: A survey of current practice, MIDIRS Midwifery Digest, 17(3): 419–522

Amitay, E.L. and Keinan-Boker, L. (2015) Breastfeeding and childhood leukaemia incidence: A meta-analysis and systematic review, *JAMA Pediatrics*, 169(6): e151025–e151025. Available online at http://archpedi.jamanetwork.com/article.aspx?articleid=2299705 (accessed 9 October 2022)

Anderson, J., Held, N. and Wright, K. (2004) Raynaud's phenomenon of the nipple: A treatable cause of nipple pain, Pediatrics, 113(4): 360–364

Asztalos, E., *et al.* (2019) Role of days post-delivery on breast milk production: A secondary analysis for the EMPOWER trial, *International Breastfeeding Journal*, 14(21). Available online at https://doi.org/10.1186%2Fs13006-019-0215-z (accessed 19 October 2022)

Avici, M., Sanlikan, F., Celik, M., *et al.* (2014) Effects of maternal obesity on antenatal, perinatal and neonatal outcomes, *The Journal of Maternal-Fetal & Neonatal Medicine*, 28(17): 2080–2083

Baby Feeding Law Group-UK (n.d.) *Current UK Laws.* Available online at www.bflg-uk.org/(accessed 9 October 2022)

Baker, P., Smith, J., Garde, A., *et al.* (2023) The political economy of infant and young child feeding: Confronting corporate power, overcoming structural barriers, and accelerating progress, *The Lancet*, 401(10375): 503–524

Ball, H. (2002) Reasons to bed-share: Why parents sleep with their infants, Journal of Reproductive and Infant Psychology, 20(4): 207–321

Ball, H. (2003) Breastfeeding, bed-sharing, and infant sleep, Birth, 30(3): 181–188

Ball, H. (2009) Bed-sharing and co-sleeping, *Perspective NCT*, 5: 10–12

Ball, H., Howel, D., Bryant, A., *et al.* (2016) Bed-sharing by breastfeeding mothers: Who bed-shares and what is the relationship with breastfeeding duration? *Acta Paediatrica*, 105: 628–634

Ball, H., Ward-Platt, M., Heslop, E., *et al.* (2006) Randomised trial of infant sleep location on the postnatal ward, Archive of Disease in Childhood, 91(12): 1005–1010

Ballard, O. and Morrow, A. (2013) Human milk composition: Nutrients and bioactive factors, *Pediatric Clinics of North America*, 60(1): 49–74. Available online at www.ncbi.nlm.nih.gov/pmc/articles/PMC3586783 (accessed 9 October 2022)

Balogun, O., O'Sullivan, E., McFadden, A., *et al.* (2016) Interventions for promoting the initiation of breastfeeding, *Cochrane Database of Systematic Review*. Available online at https://doi.org/10.1002/14651858.CD001688.pub3 (accessed 28 January 2023)

Banta-Wright, S., Shelton, K., Lowe, N., *et al.* (2012) Breast-feeding success among infants with phenylketonuria, Journal of Paediatric Nursing, 27(4): 319–327

Barrett, M., Heller, M., Fullerton Stone, H., *et al.* (2013) Raynaud phenomenon of the nipple in breastfeeding mothers, JAMA *Dermatology,*149(3): 300–306

Battersby, S. (2014) The role of the midwife in breastfeeding: Dichotomies and dissonance, British Journal of Midwifery, 22(8): 551–556

Baxter, J. (2006) Women's experience of infant feeding following birth by caesarean section, *British Journal of Midwifery*, 14(5): 290–295

Beake, S., Pellowe, C., Dykes, F., *et al.* (2011) A Systematic review of structured compared with non-structured breastfeeding programmes to support the initiation and duration of exclusive and any breastfeeding in acute and primary health care settings, *Maternal and Child Nutrition*, 8: 141–161

Bergman, J. and Bergman, N. (2014) Whose choice? Advocating birthing practices according to baby's biological needs, *The Journal of Perinatal Education,*22(1): 8–13

Bergman, N. (2019) *Birth Practices: Maternal-Neonate Separation as a Source of Toxic Stress, Birth Defects Research*. Available Online at www.kangaroula.com/wp-content/uploads/2020/02/Bergman-2019-separation-source-toxic-stress.pdf (accessed 16 October 2022)

Bergman, N., Linley, L. and Fawcus, S. (2004) Randomised control trial of skin-to-skin contact from birth versus conventional incubator for physiological stabilisation in 1200–2199 gram newborns, Acta Paediatrica, 93(6): 779–885

Bergman, N., Ludwig, R., Westrup, B., *et al.* (2019) Nurturescience versus neuroscience: A case for rethinking mother-infant behaviours and relationship, *Birth Defects Research*, 1–18

Berlo, D.K. (1960) The Process of Communication, New York: Holt, Rinehart and Winston

Berry, C., Thomas, E., Piper, K., *et al.* (2007) The histology and cytology of the human mammary gland and breastmilk, in T. Hale and P. Hartman (eds) Textbook of Human Lactation, Amarillo, TX: Hale Publishing. 35–47

Biloš, L. (2017) Polycystic ovarian syndrome and low milk supply: Is insulin resistance the missing link? *Endocrine Oncology & Metabolism*, 3(2): 49–55

Blair, P., Sidebotham, P., Evason-Coombe, C., *et al.* (2009) Hazardous co-sleeping environments and risk factors amenable to change: Case-control study of SIDS in Southwest England, *British Medical Journal*, 339: 3666. Available online at www.bmj.com/content/339/bmj.b3666.full (accessed 9 October 2022)

Blixt, I., Johansson, M., Hildingsson, I., *et al.* (2019) Women's advice to healthcare professionals regarding breastfeeding: 'Offer sensitive individualized breastfeeding support' – an interview study, *International Breastfeeding Journal*, 14(1): 51–51

Bolling, K., Grant, C., Hamlyn, B., *et al.* (2007) Infant Feeding Survey 2005, London: The Information Centre

Bompy, L., Gerenton, B., Chrisofari, S., *et al.* (2019) Impact of breastfeeding according to implant features in breast augmentation: A multicentric retrospective study, *Annals of Plastic Surgery*, 82(1): 11–14

Bortoli, J. and Amir, L. (2021) Is onset of lactation delayed in women with diabetes in pregnancy? A systematic review, *Diabetic Medicine*, 33(1): 17–24

Boswell, N. (2021) Complimentary feeding methods: A review of the benefits and risk, *International Journal of Environmental Research and Public Health*,18(13): 7165

Boud, D., Keogh, R. and Walker, D. (eds) (1985) Reflection: Turning Experience into Learning, London: Kogan Page

Bowlby, J. (1982) Attachment and Loss. Vol. 1: Attachment (2nd edn), New York: Basic Books

Breastfeeding Network (BFN) (2014) Breastfeeding if You Are on the Autistic Spectrum. Available online at www.breastfeedingnetwork.org.uk/breastfeeding-on-autistic-spectrum/ (accessed 11 December 2022)

Breastfeeding Network (BFN) (2019a) *Expressing and Storing Breast Milk*. Available online at https://www.breastfeedingnetwork.org.uk/(accessed 9 October 2022)

Breastfeeding Network (BFN) (2019b) *Creams and Ointments Applied to the Skin of Breastfeeding Mothers*. Available online at www.breastfeedingnetwork.org.uk/creams/(accessed 9 October 2022)

Breastfeeding Network (BFN) (2019c) *Smoking, Smoking Cessation and Breastfeeding*. Available online at www.breastfeedingnetwork.org.uk (accessed 9 October 2022).

Breastfeeding Network (BFN) (2019d) *Increasing Milk Supply- Use of Galactagogues*. Available online at www.breastfeedingnetwork.org.uk (accessed 18 October 2022)

Breastfeeding Network (BFN) (2020) Thrush and Breastfeeding. Available online at https://www.breastfeedingnetwork.org.uk(accessed 9 October 2022)

Breastfeeding Network (BFN) (2021) *Alcohol and Breastfeeding*. Available online at www.breastfeed ingnetwork.org.uk (accessed 9 October 2022)

Breastfeeding Network (BFN) (2022) Mastitis and Breastfeeding. Available online at www.breastfeedingnetwork.org.uk(accessed 12 January 2023)

Bridges, N. (2016) The faces of breastfeeding support: Experiences of mothers seeking breastfeeding support online, Breastfeeding Review, 24(1): 11–20

British Association of Perinatal Medicine (BAPM) (2017) *Identification and Management of Neonatal Hypoglycaemia in the Full Term Infant: A BAPM Framework for Practice*. Available online at www.bapm.org (accessed 16 October 2022)

British Association of Perinatal Medicine (BAPM) (2022) *Covid-19 Pandemic Frequently Asked Questions Within Neonatal Services*. Available online www.bapm.org (accessed 14 January 2023)

Buckley, K. (2009) A double-edged sword: Lactation consultants' perceptions of the impact of breast pumps on the practice of breastfeeding, Journal of Perinatal Education, 18(2): 13–22

Caldwell, K., Turner-Maffei, C., Blair, A., *et al.* (2004) Pain reduction and treatment of sore nipples in nursing mothers, Journal of Perinatal Education, 13(1): 29–35

Campbell-Yeo, M., Disher, T., Benoit, B., *et al.* (2015) Understanding kangaroo care and its benefits to preterm infants, *Paediatric Health Medicine*, 6: 15–32

Care Quality Commission (CQC) (2022) *Experiences of Being in Hospital for People with Learning Disability and Autistic People*. Available Online at www.cqc.org.uk (accessed 13 November 2022)

Carper, B.A. (1978) Fundamental patterns of knowing in nursing, Advances in Nursing Science, 1(1): 13–23

Cawse-Lucas, J., Waterman, S. and Leilani, A. (2015) Does frenotomy help infants with tongue-tie overcome breastfeeding difficulties? *Journal of Family Practice*, 64(2): 126–127

Channell Doig, A., Jasczynski, M., Fleishman, J.L., *et al.* (2020) Breastfeeding among mothers who have experienced childhood maltreatment: A review, *Journal of Human Lactation*, 36(4): 710–722

Charpak, N., Gabriel Ruiz, J., Zupan, J., *et al.* (2005) Kangaroo mother care: 25 years after, Acta Paediatrica, 94(5): 514–522

Chertok, I. (2009) Re-examination of ultra-thin nipple shield use, infant growth and maternal satisfaction, Journal of Clinical Nursing, 18(21): 2049–2155

Chertok, I., Raz, I., Shoham, I., *et al.* (2009) Effects of early breastfeeding on neonatal glucose levels of term infants born to women with gestational diabetes, Journal of Human Nutrition and Dietetics, 22(2): 166–169

Coentro, V., Perrella, S., Lai, C., *et al.* (2021) Impact of nipple shield use on milk transfer and maternal nipple pain, *Breastfeeding Medicine, 16*(3): 222–229

Colaizy, T., Bartick, M., Jeiger, B., *et al.* (2016) Impact of optimised breastfeeding on the costs of ne-crotizing enterocolitis in extremely low birthweight infants, *Journal of Pediatrics*, 175: 100–105

Colson, S. (2015) *Biological Nurturing: Laid Back Breastfeeding.* Available online at www.biologi-calnurturing.com/our-beliefs/ (accessed 9 October 2022)

Conde-Agudelo, A. and Díaz-Rossello, J. (2016) Kangaroo mother care to reduce morbidity and mortality in low birthweight infants, *Cochrane Database of Systematic Reviews.* Available on-line at https://doi.org/10.1002/14651858.CD002771.pub4 (accessed 19 January 2023)

Coppa, G., Bruni, S., Morelli, L., *et al.* (2004) The first prebiotics in humans: Human milk oligo-saccharides, *Journal of Clinical Gastroenterology*, 38: 80–83

Cox, D., Owens, R. and Hartmann, P. (1996) Blood and milk prolactin and the rate of milk syn-thesis in women, *Experimental Physiology*, 81: 1007–1120

Crawley, H. and Westland, S. (2017) *Baby Foods in the UK A Review of Commercially Produced Jars and Pouches of Baby Foods Marketed in the UK*, London: First Steps Nutrition Trust

Cregan, M., Mitoulas, L. and Hartmann, P. (2002) Milk prolactin, feed volume and duration between feeds in women breastfeeding their full-term infants over a 24h period, *Experimen-tal Physiology*, 87(2): 207–214. Available online at http://onlinelibrary.wiley.com/doi/10.1113/eph8702327/epdf (accessed 6 January 2023)

Crepinsek, M., Taylor, E., Michener, K., *et al.* (2020) Interventions for preventing mastitis af-ter childbirth, *Cochrane Database of Systematic Reviews.* Available online at https://doi.org/10.1002/14651858.CD007239.pub4 (accessed 8 January 2023)

Czank, C., Henderson, J., Kent, J., *et al.* (2007a) Hormonal control of the lactation cycle, in T. Hale and P. Hartmann (eds) Textbook of Human Lactation, Amarillo, TX: Hale Publishing. 89–112

Czank, C., Mitoulas, L.R. and Hartmann, P. (2007b) Human milk composition: Fat, in T. Hale and P. Hartmann (eds) Textbook of Human Lactation, Amarillo, TX: Hale Publishing. 49–68

D'Andrea, M. and Spatz, D. (2019) Maintaining breastfeeding during severe infant and maternal HSV-1 infection: A case report, *Journal of Human Lactation*, 35(4). Available online at https://doi-org.knowledge.idm.oclc.org/10.1177/0890334419830994 (accessed 13 January 2023)

Dayal, D., Soni, V., Jayaraman, D., *et al.* (2016) Cultural gynecomastia in the 21st century India: 'Witch's milk revisited'. *Pediatria Polska* 91: 472–475

Dennis, C., Jackson, K. and Watson, J. (2014) Interventions for treating painful nipples among breastfeeding women, *Cochrane Database of Systematic Reviews.* Available online at https://doi.org/10.1002/14651858.CD007366.pub2 (accessed 12 January 2023)

Department of Health and Social Care (DHSC) (2016) *Childhood Obesity: A Plan for Action.* Available online at www.gov.uk(accessed 1 October 2022)

Department of Health and Social Care (DHSC) (2017) *Drug Misuse and Dependence: UK Guide-lines on Clinical Management.* Available online at www.gov.uk (accessed 15 January 2023)

Department of Health and Social Care (DHSC) (2020) *Tackling Obesity: Empowering Adults and Children to Live Healthier Lives.* Available online at www.gov.uk (accessed 1 October 2022)

Department of Health and Social Care (DHSC) (2022) *New Campaign Promotes Advice to Intro-duce Babies to Solid Food.* Available online at www.gov.uk (accessed 9 October 2022)

Dewey, K., Nommsen-Rivers, L. and Heinig, J. (2005) Risk factors for suboptimal infant breast-feeding behaviour, delayed onset of lactogenesis, and excessive neonatal weight loss, *Pediatrics*, 112: 607–619

Dickens, V. (2008) Learning on the job: Influences on the initiation and duration of breastfeeding, MIDIRS Midwifery Digest, 18(2): 243–247

Dixon, K., Ferris, R., Marikar, D., *et al.* (2017) Definition and monitoring of neonatal hypoglycaemia: A nationwide survey of NHS England neonatal units, *Archives of Disease in Childhood*, 102(1): 92–93

Dogan, E., Yilmaz, C., Turgut, M., *et al.* (2018) Baby-led complementary feeding: Randomised controlled study, *Pediatrics International*, 60(12): 1073–1080

Dorea, J. (2007) Maternal smoking and infant feeding: Breastfeeding is better and safer, *Maternal and Child Health*, 11: 287–391

Doughty, K. and Taylor, S. (2021) Barriers and benefits to breastfeeding with gestational diabetes, *Seminars in Perinatology*, 45(2). Available online at https://doi-org.knowledge.idm.oclc.org/10.1016/j.semperi.2020.151385 (accessed 12 January 2023)

Douglas, P. (2022) Re-thinking benign inflammation of the lactating breast: Classification, prevention and management, *Women's Health*, 18. Available online at https://doi.org/10.1177/17455057221091349 (accessed 13 January 2023)

Dryden, C., Young, D., Hepburn, M., *et al.* (2009) Maternal methadone use in pregnancy: Factors associated with the development of neonatal abstinence syndrome and implications for healthcare resources, *British Journal of Obstetrics and Gynaecology*, 116: 665–671

Dykes, F. (2003) Protecting and supporting breastfeeding, British Journal of Midwifery, 11(10): 24–48

Dyson, L., Renfrew, M., McFadden, A., *et al.* (2006) Promotion of Initiation and Duration of Breastfeeding: Evidence into Practice Briefing, London: NICE

Eagen-Torkko, M., Low, L., Zielinski, R., *et al.* (2017) Prevalence and predictors of breastfeeding after childhood abuse, *Journal of Obstetric, Gynecologic, & Neonatal Nursing*, 46(3): 465–479

East, C., Dolan, W. and Forster, D. (2014) Antenatal breast milk expression by women with diabetes for improving infant outcomes, *Cochrane Database of Systematic Reviews*. Available online at https://doi.org/10.1002/14651858.CD010408.pub2 (accessed 15 January 2023)

Eglash, A. (2014) Treatment of maternal hypergalactia, *Breastfeeding Medicine*, 9(9): 423–425

Employment Rights Act (1996) London: HMSO. Available online at https://www.legislation.gov.uk/ukpga/1996/18/contents (accessed 16 April 2023)

Entwistle, F. (2013) The Evidence and Rationale for the UNICEF UK Baby Friendly Initiative Standards, London: UNICEF Baby Friendly UK

Equality Act (2010) London: HMSO. Available online at https://www.legislation.gov.uk/ukpga/2010/15/contents (accessed 13 April 2023)

Fangupo, L., Heath, A., Williams, S., *et al.* (2016) A baby-led approach to eating solids and risk of choking, *Pediatrics*, 138(4): e20160772

Fawcett, J., Watson, J., Neuman, B., *et al.* (2001) On nursing theories and evidence, *Journal of Nursing Scholarship*, 33: 115–119. Available online at https://doi.org/10.1111/j.1547-5069.2001.00115.x (accessed 24 January 2023)

Finigan, V. (2009) 'It's on the tip of my tongue': Evaluation of a new frenulotomy service in northern England, MIDIRS Midwifery Digest, 19(3): 395–400

Fitzgerald, E., Hor, K. and Drake, A. (2020) Maternal influences on fetal brain development: The role of nutrition, infection and stress, and the potential for intergenerational consequences, *Early Human Development*, 50. Available online at www.sciencedirect.com/science/article/pii/S0378378220306514 (accessed 9 October 2022)

Flint, A., New, K. and Davies, M. (2016) Cup feeding versus other forms of supplemental enteral feeding for newborn infants unable to fully breastfeed, *Cochrane Database of Systematic Reviews*. Available online at https://doi.org/10.1002/14651858.CD005092.pub3 (accessed 22 January 2023)

Food Standards Agency (FSA) (2013) *Committee on Toxicity of Chemicals in Food, Consumer Products and the Environment*. Available online at https://cot.food.gov.uk/sites/default/files/cot/tox201315.pdf (accessed 22 January2023)

Food Standards Agency (FSA) (2018) *An Investigation into the Attitudes and Behaviours of Consumers and Caregivers in the Preparation, Handling and Storage and Feeding of Powdered*

Infant Formula Inside and Outside the Home. Available online at www.food.gov.uk/ (accessed 28 October 2022)

Food Standards Agency (FSA) (2021) *Committee on Toxicity of Chemicals in Food, Consumer Products and the Environment. Overarching Statement on Consumption of Plant-based Drinks in Children Aged 6 Months to 5 Years.* Available online at https://cot.food.gov.uk/2021-stateme ntsandpositionpapers(accessed 28 October 2022)

Foong, S., Marasco, L., Ho, J., *et al.* (2020) Oral galactagogues (natural therapies or drugs) for increasing breastmilk production in mothers of non-hospitalised term infants, *Cochrane Database of Systematic Reviews.* Available online at https://doi.org/10.1002/14651858.CD011505.pub2 (accessed 18 October 2022)

Forster, D., Moorhead, A., Jacobs, S., *et al.* (2017) Advising women with diabetes in pregnancy to express breastmilk in late pregnancy (diabetes and antenatal milk expressing [DAME]): A multicentre, unblinded, randomised control trial, *Lancet, 389:* 2204–2213

Foster, J., Psaila, K. and Patterson, T. (2016) Non-nutritive sucking for increasing physiologic stability and nutrition in preterm infants, *Cochrane Database of Systematic Reviews.* Available online at https://doi.org/10.1002/14651858.CD001071.pub3 (accessed 19 January 2022)

Frazier, D., Allgeier, C., Homer, C., *et al.* (2014) Nutrition management guideline for maple syrup urine disease: An evidence- and consensus-based approach, Molecular Genetics and Metabolism, 112(3): 210–217

Gavine, A., MacGillivray, S., Renfrew, M., *et al.* (2016) Education and training of healthcare staff in the knowledge, attitudes and skills needed to work effectively with breastfeeding women: A systematic review, *International Breastfeeding Journal,* 12(6). Available online at www.ncbi.nlm. nih.gov/pmc/articles/PMC5288894 (accessed 9 October 2022)

Gavine, A., Shimwell., Bucchan, P., *et al.* (2022) Support for healthy breastfeeding mothers with healthy term babies, *Cochrane Database of Systematic Reviews.* Available online at https://doi. org/10.1002/14651858.CD001141.pub6 (accessed 4 January 2023)

Geddes, D. (2007a) Inside the lactating breast: The latest anatomy research, Journal of Midwifery and Women's Health, 52(6): 556–663

Geddes, D. (2007b) Gross anatomy of the lactating breast, in T. Hale and P. Hartmann (eds) Textbook of Human Lactation, Amarillo, TX: Hale Publishing. 19–34

Geddes, D., Gridneva, Z., Perella, S., *et al.* (2021) 25 Years of research in human lactation: From discovery to translation, *Nutrients,* 8(12). Available online at www.mdpi.com/2072-6643/13/9/3071/htm (accessed 10 October 2022)

Geddes, D., Langton, D. and Gallow, I. (2008) Frenulotomy for breastfeeding infants with ankyloglossia: Effect on milk removal and sucking mechanism as imaged by ultrasound, Pediatrics, 122(1): 188–294

Gibbs, G. (1998) Learning by Doing: A Guide to Teaching and Learning Methods, London: Further Education Unit

Giglia, R., Binns, C. and Alfonso, H. (2006) Maternal cigarette smoking and breastfeeding duration, *Acta Paediatrica,* 95: 1370–1374

The Global Breastfeeding Collective (2017) *Global Breastfeeding Scorecard, The Global Breastfeeding Collective.* Available online at www.globalbreastfeedingcollective.org/ (accessed 9 October 2022)

Graignic-Philippe, R., Dayan, J., Chokron, S., *et al.* (2014) Effects of prenatal stress on fetal and child development: A critical literature review, *Neuroscience & Biobehavioral Reviews,* 43: 137–162

Gray, J. (2001) Evidence-Based Health Care (2nd edn), London: Churchill Livingstone.

Gregson, S., Meadows, J., Teakle, P., *et al.* (2016) Skin-to-skin contact after elective caesarean section: Investigating the effect on breastfeeding rates. British Journal of Midwifery, 24(1): 18–25

Grove, S., Gray, J. and Burns, N. (2014) Understanding Nursing Research: Building an Evidence-Based Practice (6th edn), Missouri: Elsevier Saunders.

Grummer-Strawn, L. and Rollins, N. (2015) Summarising the health effects of breastfeeding, *ACTA Paediatrica,* 104(S467): 1–2

Güemes, M., Rahman, S. and Hussain, K. (2016) What is normal blood glucose? *Archives of Disease in Childhood*, 101(6): 569–574

Habron, J., Booley, S., Najaar, B., *et al.* (2013) Responsive feeding: Establishing healthy eating behaviour early on in life, South African Journal of Clinical Nutrition, 26(3): 141–149

Hake-Brooks, S. and Anderson, G. (2008) Kangaroo care and breastfeeding of mother – preterm infant dyads 0–18 months: A randomised controlled trial, *Neonatal Network*, 27: 151–159

Han, S. and Hong, Y. (1999) The inverted nipple: Its grading and surgical correction, *Plastic Reconstructive Surgery*, 104: 389–395

Handlin, L., Jonas, W., Peterson, M., *et al.* (2009) Effects of sucking and skin-to-skin contact on maternal ACTH and cortisol levels during the second day postpartum: influence of epidural analgesia and oxytocin in the perinatal period, Breastfeed Med, 4(4): 207–220

Harding, C. (2009) An evaluation of the benefits of non-nutritive sucking for premature infants as described in the literature, Archives of Disease in Childhood, 94(8): 636–740

Hartmann, P. and Ramsay, D. (2006) Mammary anatomy and physiology, in E. Jones and C. King (eds) Feeding and Nutrition in the Preterm Infant, London: Elsevier

Heath, H. (1998) Reflection and patterns of knowing in nursing, *Journal of Advanced Nursing*, 27: 1054–1059

Henderson, J., Hartmann, P. and Newham, J. (2008) Effects of preterm birth and antenatal corticosteroid treatment on lactogenesis II in women, *Pediatrics*, 121: 92–100

Henry, L. and Britz, S. (2013) Loss of blood=loss of breastmilk? The effect of postpartum hemorrhage on breastfeeding success, *Journal of Obstetric, Gynecological & Neonatal Nursing*, 42(1). Available online at https://doi.org/10.1111/1552-6909.12198 (accessed 18 January 2023)

Hepatitis B Foundation (2020) *Pregnancy and Hepatitis B*. Available online at www.hepb.org(accessed 29 January 2023)

Herron, M., Sinclair, M., Kernohan, W.G., *et al.* (2015) Tapping into authentic presence: Key components arising from a concept analysis of online breastfeeding support, Evidence Based Midwifery, 13(3): 76–83

Hersh, C., Sorbo, J., Moreno, J., *et al.* (2022) Aspiration does not mean the end of breastfeeding relationship, *International Journal of Pediatric Otorhinolaryngology*, 161. Available online https://doi.org/10.1016/j.ijporl.2022.111263 (accessed 25 October 2022)

Hewitt, H. (2008) Peer influence, MIDIRS Midwifery Digest, 18(2): 260–262

Hilton, S. (2008) Milk production during pregnancy and beyond, British Journal of Midwifery, 16(8): 544–548

Hogan, M., Westcott, C. and Griffiths, M. (2005) Randomised control trial of division of tongue-tie in infants with feeding problems, Journal of Paediatrics and Child Health, 41(5–6): 246–350

Homeyard, C. and Patelarou, E. (2018) To what extent are midwives adapting antenatal information for pregnant women with intellectual disabilities? A survey of NHS trusts in England, *Public Health*, 158: 25–30

Horta, B., Matrinés, J., Victora, C., *et al.* (2007) *Evidence on the Long-Term Effects of Breastfeeding*, Geneva: WHO

Horta, B. and Victora, C. (2013) *Long-Term Effects of Breastfeeding: A Systematic Review*, Geneva: WHO

Howatson-Jones, L. (2016) Reflective Practice in Nursing, London: Sage Publications

Hurley, K., Cross, M. and Hughes, S. (2011) A systematic review of responsive feeding and child obesity in high-income countries, Journal of Nutrition, 141(3): 1–7

Hurst, N. (2007) Recognising and treating delayed or failed lactogenesis II, Journal of Midwifery & Women's Health, 52(6): 588–694

Ingram, J., Johnson, D. and Condon, L. (2011) The effects of Baby Friendly Initiative training on breastfeeding attitudes, knowledge and self-efficacy of community healthcare staff, *Primary Health Care Research & Development*, 12: 266–275

Ingram, J., Thomson, G., Johnson, D., *et al.* (2020) Women's and peer supporters' experiences of an assets-based peer support intervention for increasing breastfeeding initiation and continuation: A qualitative study, *Health Expectations*, 23(3): 622–631

Inherited Metabolic Disorders in Scotland (IMD Scotland) (2017) *Metabolic Conditions*. Available online at www.imd.scot.nhs.uk (accessed 25 October 2022)

Ip, S., Raman, G., Chew, P., *et al.* (2007) *Breastfeeding and Maternal Health Outcomes in Developed Countries: Evidence Report/Technology Assessment No. 153*, Agency for Healthcare Research and Quality. Available online at http://archive.ahrq.gov/downloads/pub/evidence/pdf/brfout/brfout.pdf (accessed 9 October 2022)

Islam, M. (2016) Why are 'hard-to-reach' women not engaging in breastfeeding support programmes? Community Practitioner, 89(2): 36–41

Iyer, N., Srinivasan, R., Evans, K., *et al.* (2008) Impact of early weighing policy on neonatal hypernatraemic dehydration and breastfeeding, Archives of Childhood Disease, 93(4): 297–299

Jaafar, S., Ho, J., Jahanfar, S., *et al.* (2016a) Effect of restricted pacifier use in breastfeeding term infants for increasing duration of breastfeeding, *Cochrane Database of Systematic Reviews*. Available online at https://doi.org/10.1002/14651858.CD007202.pub4 (accessed 22 January 2023)

Jaafar, S., Ho, J. and Lee, K. (2016b) Rooming-in for new mother and infant versus separate care for increasing the duration of breastfeeding, *Cochrane Library, Cochrane Database of Systematic Reviews*. Available online at https://doi.org/10.1002/14651858.CD006641.pub3 (accessed 29 January 2023)

Jackson, W. (2004) Breastfeeding and type 1 diabetes mellitus, British Journal of Midwifery, 12(3): 158–265

Jambert-Gray, R., Lucas, K. and Hall, V. (2009) Methadone-treated mothers: Pregnancy and breastfeeding, British Journal of Midwifery, 17(10): 654–657

Januszewski, A. (2001) Educational Technology: The Development of a Concept, Santa Barbara, CA: Libraries Unlimited Inc

Joham, A., Nanayakkara, N., Ranasinha, S., *et al.* (2016) Obesity, polycystic ovary syndrome and breastfeeding: An observational study, *Acta Obstetrica et Gynecologica Scandinavica*, 95(4): 458–466. Available online at https://doi.org/10.1111/aogs.12850 (accessed 18 January 2023)

Johns, C. (1995) Framing learning through reflection within Carper's fundamental ways of knowing in nursing, *Journal of Advanced Nursing*, 22: 226–334

Johnson, C., *et al.* (2021) Supporting women with learning disabilities in infant feeding decisions: A scoping review, *Maternal & Child Nutrition*, 18: e13318

Johnston, C., Filion, F. and Campbell-Yeo, M. (2008) Kangaroo mother care diminishes pain from heel lance in very preterm infants: A cross-over trial, MIDIRS Midwifery Digest, 18(4): 574–575

Jonas, W., Nissen, E., Ransjö-Arvidson, A., *etal.* (2008) Short- and long-term decrease of blood pressure in women during breastfeeding, Breastfeed Medicine, 3: 103–109

Jones, E. and Spencer, S. (2008) Optimising the provision of human milk in preterm infants, MIDIRS Midwifery Digest, 18(1): 118–221

Karlsson, J., Garnett, T., Rollins, N., *et al.* (2019) The carbon footprint of breastmilk substitutes in comparison with breastmilk, *Journal of Cleaner Production*, 222: 436–445

Katz, J., Lee, A. and Kozuki, N. (2013) Mortality risk in preterm and small-for-gestational-age infants in low-income and middle-income countries: A pooled country analysis, The Lancet, 382(9890): 417–525

Kaunonen, M., Hannula, L. and Tarkka, M.J. (2012) A systematic review of peer support interventions for breastfeeding, *Journal of Clinical Nursing*, 21: 1943–1954

Keely, A., Lawton, J., Swanson, V., *et al.* (2015) Barriers to breastfeeding in obese women: A qualitative exploration, *Midwifery*, 31(5): 532–539

Kendall-Tackett, K. (2017) Why trauma-informed care needs to be the standard of care for IB-CLCs, *Clinical Lactation*, 8(4): 150–152

Kent, J. (2007) How breastfeeding works, Journal of Midwifery & Women's Health, 52(6): 564–670

Kent, J., Ashton, E., Hardwick, C., *et al.* (2015) Nipple pain in breastfeeding mothers: Incidence, causes and treatments, *International Journal of Environmental Research and Public Health*, 12(10): 12247–12263

Kent, J., Gardner, H. and Geddes, D. (2016) Breastmilk production in the first 4 weeks after birth of term infants, *Nutrients, 8(12): 756

Kent, J., Mitoulas, L., Cregan, M., *et al.* (2006) Volume and frequency of breastfeeding and fat content of breastmilk throughout the day, Pediatrics, 117(3): 387–395

Kent, J., Mitoulas, L., Cregan, M., *etal.* (2008) Importance of vacuum for breastmilk expression, *Breastfeed Medicine*, 3: 11–19

Khajehei, M., Doherty, M., Tilley, P.J., *et al.* (2015) Prevalence and risk factors of sexual dysfunction in postpartum Australian women, *The Journal of Sexual Medicine*, 12(6): 1415–1426

Kim, S. and Yi, D. (2020) Components of human breast milk: From macronutrient to microbiome and microRNA, Pediatrics, 63(8): 301–309

Knight, C., Peaker, M. and Wilde, C. (1998) Local control of mammary development and function, *Reviews of Reproduction*, 3: 104–212

Kramer, M., Aboud, F. and Mironova, E. (2008) Breastfeeding and child cognitive development: New evidence from a large randomised trial, *Archives of General Psychiatry*, 65: 578–684

Krogstad, P., Contreras, D., Ng, H., *et al.* (2022) No infectious SARS-CoV-2 in breast milk from a cohort of 110 lactating women, *Pediatric Research*, 92: 1140–1145

Kronborg, H., Vaeth, M., Olsen, O., *etal.* (2007) Health visitors and breastfeeding support: Influence of knowledge and self-efficacy, European Journal of Public Health, 18(3): 283–288

Kruger, E., Kritzinger, A. and Pottas, L. (2019) Oropharyngeal dysplasia in breastfeeding neonates with hypoxic-ischaemic encephalopathy on therapeutic hypothermia, *Breastfeed Med*, 14(10): 718–723

Ladhani, S., Srinivasan, L., Buchanan, C., *et al.* (2004) Presentation of vitamin D deficiency, *Archives of Disease in Childhood*, 89: 781–784

Law, C., Wolfenden, L., Sperlich, M., *et al.* (2021) *A Good Practice Guide to Support Implementation of Trauma-informed Care in the Perinatal Period*, Blackpool: The Centre for Early Child Development

Letourneau, N., Waton, B., Duffet-Legger, L., *etal.* (2011) Cortisol patterns of depressed mothers and their infants are related to maternal – infant interactive behaviours, Journal of Reproductive and Infant Psychology, 29(5): 439–459

Levene, M., Tudehope, D. and Sinha, S. (2008) Essential Neonatal Medicine (4th edn), London: Blackwell

LGBT Foundation (2022) *Trans and Non-Binary Experiences of Maternity Services.* Available online at www.lgbt.foundation/ (accessed 15 July 2022)

Li, L., Wan, W. and Zhu, C. (2021) Breastfeeding after a caesarean section: A literature review, *Midwifery, 103.* Available online at https://doi.org/10.1016/j.midw.2021.103117 (accessed 29 November 2022)

Linnecar, A., Gupta, A., Dadhich, J., *etal.* (2014) Formula for Disaster: Weighing the Impact of Formula Feeding vs Breastfeeding on Environment, Delhi: BPNI/IBFAN

Liu, B., Beral, V. and Balkwall, A. (2009) Childbearing, breastfeeding, other reproductive factors and the subsequent risk of hospitalization for gallbladder disease, *International Journal of Epidemiology*, 38(1): 312–318. Available online at http://ije.oxfordjournals.org/content/early/2008/09/04/ije.dyn174.short (accessed 9 October 2022)

Livingstone, V. (1996) Too much of a good thing: Maternal and infant hyperlactation syndromes, *Canadian Family Physician*, 42: 89–99

Livingstone, V., Willis, C., Abdel-Wareth, L., *et al.* (2000) Neonatal hypernatraemic dehydration, Canadian Medical Association Journal, 162(5): 647–652

Lommens, A., Brown, B. and Hollist, D. (2013) Experiential perceptions of relactation. A phenomenological study, Journal of Human Lactation, 21(3): 109–112

Lubbe, W. and ten Ham-Baloyi, W. (2017) When is the use of pacifiers justifiable in the baby-friendly hospital initiative context? A clinician's guide, *BMC Pregnancy & Childbirth*, 17: 130

Lubbers, C. (1990) Communication skills for continuing education in nursing, Journal of Continuing Education in Nursing, 21(3): 109–212

Lullaby Trust (2022) *How to Reduce the Risk of SIDS.* Available online at www.lullabytrust.org.uk (accessed 29 January 2023)

Lumbiganon, P., Martis, R., Laopaiboon, M., *etal.* (2016) Antenatal breastfeeding education for increasing breastfeeding duration, *Cochrane Database of Systematic Reviews*. Available online at https://doi.org/10.1002/14651858.CD006425.pub4 (accessed 5 January 2023)

Mansoori, M. and Salmani, N. (2020) Effect of breast milk expression during kangaroo mother care on milk volume in mothers with premature infants admitted to neonatal intensive care unit, *Evidence Based Care Journal*, 10(1): 44–50

Marks, D. and O'Connor, R. (2015) Health professionals' attitudes towards the promotion of breastfeeding, British Journal of Midwifery, 23(1): 854–962

Martin, C., Ling, P.R. and Blackburn, G. (2016) Review of infant feeding: Key features of breast-milk and infant formula, *Nutrients*, 8(5): 279

Martyn, T. (2003) Infant feeding, Midwives, 6(5): 215

Matthiesen, A., Ransjö-Arvidson, A., Nissen, E., *et al.* (2001) Postpartum maternal oxytocin release by newborns: effects of infant hand massage and sucking, Birth, 28(1): 20–21

McAndrew, F., Thomson, J., Fellows, L., *et al.* (2012) Infant Feeding Survey 2010, Leeds: Health and Social Care Information Centre

McCrory, F. and Richens, Y. (2007) Pregnancy, parenting and substance misuse, in Y. Richens (ed) Challenges for Midwives Volume II, London: Quay Books. 201–213

McFadden, A., Renfrew, M.J., Wallace, L., *et al.* (2007) Does breastfeeding really matter? A National multidisciplinary breastfeeding knowledge and skills assessment, MIDIRS Midwifery Digest, 17(1): 85–88

McGrath, J. and Braescu, A. (2004) State of the science feeding readiness in the preterm infant, Journal of Perinatal and Neonatal Nursing, 18(4): 353–470

McInnes, R. and Chambers, J. (2006) Breastfeeding in Neonatal Units: A Review of Breastfeeding Publications between 1990–2005, Edinburgh: NHS Health Scotland/Scottish Executive.

McInnes, R. and Chambers, J. (2008a) Infants admitted to neonatal units – interventions to improve breastfeeding outcomes: A systematic review 1990–2007, *Maternal and Child Health*, 4: 235–363

McInnes, R. and Chambers, J. (2008b) Supporting breastfeeding mothers: Qualitative synthesis, Journal of Advanced Nursing, 62(4): 407–527

McKinney, C., Glass, R. and Coffey, P. (2016) Feeding neonates by cup: A systematic review of the literature, Maternal and Child Health Journal, 20(8): 1620–1633

Mencap (2022) *How Common is Learning Disability*? Available Online at www.mencap.org.uk/learning-disability-explained (accessed 13 November 2022)

Menella, J. and Pepino, M. (2008) Biphasic effects of moderate drinking on prolactin during lactation, Alcoholism: Clinical and Experimental Research, 32(11): 1899–1908

Mitchell, J., Jones, W., Winkley, E., *et al.* (2020) Guideline on anaesthesia and sedation in breastfeeding women, *Anaesthesia*, 75(11): 1482–1493

Moberg, K. (2003) The Oxytocin Factor: Tapping the Hormone of Calm, Loving and Healing, Cambridge, MA: Da Capo Press

Mohd Hassan, S., Sulaiman, Z. and Tengku Ismail, T. (2021) Experienced of women who underwent induced lactation: A literature review, *Malaysian Family Physician*, 16(1): 18–30

Moore, E., Anderson, G., Bergman, N., *et al.* (2012) Early skin-to-skin contact for mothers and their healthy newborn infants, *Cochrane Database of Systematic Reviews*. Available online at https://doi.org/10.1002/14651858.CD003519.pub3 (accessed 19 January 2023)

Moore, E., Anderson, G., Bergman, N., *et al.* (2016) Early skin-to-skin contact for mothers and their healthy newborn infants, *Cochrane Database of Systematic Reviews*. Available online at https://doi.org/10.1002/14651858.CD003519.pub4 (accessed 5 January 2023)

Moser, K., Whittle, C. and Hicks, C. (2003) Social inequalities in low birth weight in England and Wales: Trends and implications for future population health, *Journal of Epidemiology and Community Health*, 57: 687–791

Napierala, M., Mazela, J., Merritt, T., *et al.* (2016) Tobacco smoking and breastfeeding: Effect on the lactation process, breast milk composition and infant development. A critical review, *Environmental Research*, 151: 321–338

National Institute for Health and Clinical Excellence (NICE) (2010) Donor Milk Banks: Nice Clinical Guideline CG93. Available online at www.nice.org.uk/guidance/cg93 (accessed 22 January 2023)

National Institute for Health and Clinical Excellence (NICE) (2011) Division of Ankyloglossia (Tongue-Tie) for Breastfeeding (Shared Learning Database), London: NICE

National Institute for Health and Clinical Excellence (NICE) (2016) *Jaundice in the Newborn*, London: NICE

National Institute for Health and Clinical Excellence (NICE) (2017) *Faltering Growth: Recognition and Management of Faltering Growth in Children: Nice Clinical Guideline 75*, London: NICE

National Institute for Health and Clinical Excellence (NICE) (2018a) *Social and Emotional Wellbeing: Early Years (updated from 2012)*, London: NICE

National Institute for Health and Clinical Excellence (NICE) (2018b) *Faltering Growth: Weight Loss in the First Few Days after Birth*, London: NICE. Available online at https://cks.nice.org.uk/topics/faltering-growth/management/weight-loss-in-the-first-few-days-after-birth/ (accessed 29 November 2022)

National Institute for Health and Clinical Excellence (NICE) (2021a) *Postnatal Care, NCGUNICEUNICEF 194*, London: NICE

National Institute for Health and Clinical Excellence (NICE) (2021b) *Mastitis and Breast Abscess*. Available online at https://cks.nice.org.uk/topics/mastitis-breast-abscess/management/management-lactating-women (accessed 9 October 2022)

National Institute for Health and Clinical Excellence (NICE) (2022a) *Scenario: Breastfeeding Problems- Management*. Available online at Scenario: Breastfeeding problems – management | Management | Breastfeeding problems | CKS | NICE (accessed 12 January 2023)

National Institute for Health and Clinical Excellence (NICE) (2022b) *Epilepsy*. Available online at https://bnf.nice.org.uk/treatment-summaries/epilepsy (accessed 18 January 2023)

National Institute on Drug Abuse (NIDA) (2020) *Substance Use While Pregnant and Breastfeeding*. Available online at www.drugabuse.gov/publications/research-reports/substance-use-in-women/substance-use-while-pregnant-breastfeeding (accessed 9 October 2022)

NHS (2018) *Drinks and Cups for Babies and Young Children*. Available online at www.nhs.uk (accessed 18 September 2022)

NHS (2019a) *Types of Formula*. Available online at www.nhs.uk (accessed 18 September 2022)

NHS (2019b) *Weaning and Feeding*. Available online at www.nhs.uk (accessed 8 August 2022)

NHS (2020) *Vitamin D: Vitamins and Minerals*. Available online at www.nhs.uk/(accessed 27 October 2022)

NHS (2022) *Breastfeeding and Drinking Alcohol*. Available online at www.nhs.uk/(accessed 15 January 2023)

NHS Health Scotland (2016) Breastfeeding and Returning to Work, Edinburgh: Health Scotland

Nickell, W. and Skelton, J. (2005) Breast fat and fallacies, Journal of Human Lactation, 21(2): 126–230

Nissen, E., Uvnas-Moberg, K., Svensson, K., *et al.* (1996) Different patterns of oxytocin, prolactin but not cortisol release during breastfeeding in women delivered by Caesarean section or by the vaginal route, *Early Human Development*, 45: 103–118

Noble, L. and Rosen-Carole, C. (2022) Breastfeeding infants with problems, in R. Lawrence and R. Lawrence (eds) Breastfeeding: A Guide for the Medical Profession (9th edn), Philadelphia: Elsevier

Nommsen-Rivers, L., Heinig, M., Cohen, R., *etal.* (2008) Newborn wet and soiled diaper counts and timing of onset of lactation as indicators of breastfeeding inadequacy, *Journal of Human Lactation*, 24: 27–33.

Nuffield Trust (2022) *Evidence for Better Health*. Available online at www.nuffieldtrust.org.uk/resource/obesity (accessed 1 October 2022)

Nursing and Midwifery Council (NMC) (2015) The Code: Professional Standards of Practice and Behaviour for Nurses and Midwives (Updated 2018), London: NMC

Nursing and Midwifery Council (NMC) (2018) *Future Nurse: Standards of Proficiency for Registered Nurses*, London: NMC

Nursing and Midwifery Council (NMC) (2019) *Standards of Proficiency for Midwives*, London: NMC

O'Brien, M., Buikstra, E., Fallon, T., *et al.* (2009) Strategies for success: A toolbox of coping strategies used by breastfeeding women, *Journal of Clinical Nursing*, 18: 1574–1582

Office for Health Improvement Disparities (OHID) (2022a) *Better Health Start for Life Weaning Campaign*. London: OHID

Office for Health Improvement Disparities (OHID) (2022b) *Small Area Associations between Breastfeeding and Obesity*, London: OHID

Oot, L., Mason, F. and Lapping, K. (2021) The first food system: The importance of breastfeeding in global systems discussions. *Global Policy Brief*. Available online at http://resource-centre-uploads.s3.amazonaws.com/uploads/sc_fhi_solutions_alivethrive_breastfeeding_and_food_systems_brief.pdf (accessed 29 May 2022)

Osborn, D. and Sinn, J. (2013) Prebiotics in infants for prevention of allergy, *Cochrane Database of Systematic Reviews*. Available online at https://doi.org/10.1002/14651858.CD006474.pub3 (accessed 27 October 2022)

O'Shea, J., Foster, J., O'Donnell, C., *et al.* (2017) Frenotomy for tongue-tie in newborn infants, *Cochrane Database of Systematic Reviews*. Available online at https://doi.org/10.1002/14651858.CD011065.pub2 (accessed 27 October 2022)

Osman, A., Celik, M. and Samanci, S. (2021) Evaluation of term newborn patients with hypernatremic dehydration, *Turkish Archives of Pediatrics*, 56(4): 344–349

Paley, J., Cheyne, H., Dalgleish, L., *et al.* (2007) Nursing's ways of knowing and dual process theories of cognition, Journal of Advanced Nursing, 60(6): 692–701

Palmer, G. (2017) *Why the of Politics Breastfeeding Matter*, London: Pinter and Martin

Parahoo, K. (2014) Nursing Research: Principles, Process and Issues (3rd edn), Basingstoke: Palgrave MacMillan

Parker, L., Sullivan., Mueller, M., *et al.* (2012) Effect of early breast milk expression on milk volume and timing of lactogenesis stage II among mothers of very low birth weight infants: A pilot study, *Journal of Perinatology*, 32: 205–209

Penny, F., Judge, M., Brownell, E., *et al.* (2018) Cup feeding as a supplemental, alternative feeding method for preterm breastfed infants: An integrative review, *Maternal and Child Health Journal*, 22: 1568–1579

Pérez-Escamilla, R., Tomori, C., Hernández-Cordero, S., *et al.* (2023) Breastfeeding: Crucially important, but increasingly challenged in a market-driven world, *The Lancet*, 401(10375): 472–485

Pikwer, M., Bergström, U., Nilsson, J., *et al.* (2008) Breastfeeding, but not oral contraceptives, is associated with a reduced risk of rheumatoid arthritis, *Annals of the Rheumatic Diseases*, 68: 526–530. Available online at http://ard.bmj.com/content/early/2008/05/13/ard.2007.084707.abstract (accessed 27 October 2022)

Pollard, M. (2010) *Learning about Breastfeeding in a Baby Friendly Accredited Pre-Registration Midwifery Programme*, unpublished EdD thesis, University of Strathclyde

Pollard, M. (2023 in press) The breasts and lactation, in: J. Rankin (ed) Physiology in Childbearing (4th edn), London: Elsevier

Preusting, I., Brumley, J. and Louis, J. (2017) Obesity as a predictor of delayed lactogenesis ll, *Journal of Human Lactation*, 33(4), 684–691

Price, E., Weaver, G., Hoffman, P., *et al.* (2016) Decontamination of breast pump milk collection kits and related items at home and in hospital: Guidance from a joint working group of the healthcare infection society and infection prevention society. *Journal of Hospital Infection*, 92: 213–221

Prior, V. and Glaser, D. (2006) Understanding Attachment and Attachment Disorders: Theory, Evidence and Practice, London: Jessica Kingsley Publishers

Public Health Agency (PHA) (2022) Off to a Good Start, Belfast: PHA

Public Health England (PHE) (2019) Pregnancy and Tuberculosis. Information for Clinicians, London: PHE

Public Health Scotland (PHS) (2021) *Formula Feeding. How to Feed Your Baby Safely*. Available online at www.healthscotland.com/ (accessed 28 October 2022)

Public Health Scotland (PHS) (2022) *Fun First Foods*. Available online at www.healthscotland.com/ (accessed 28 October 2022)

Quigley, M., Embleton, N. and McGuire, W. (2019) Formula versus donor breast milk for feeding preterm or low birth weight infants, *Cochrane Database of Systematic Reviews*. Available online at https://doi.org/10.1002/14651858.CD002971.pub5 (accessed 22 January 2023)

Raina, A. and Preston, N. (2014) Human immunodeficiency virus and infant feeding, Infant, 10(1): 5–8

Ramsay, D., Kent, J., Hartmann, R., *et al.* (2005) Anatomy of the lactating breast redefined with ultrasound imaging, Journal of Anatomy, 206(6): 525–534

Rapley, G. (2008) *Baby-led Weaning*. Available online at www.rapleyweaning.com/leaflets.php (accessed 22 January 2023)

Rapley, G. (2011) Baby-led weaning: Transitioning to solid foods at baby's own pace, Community Practitioner, 84(6): 20–23

Rasmussen, K. and Kjolhede, C. (2004) Pre-pregnant overweight and obesity diminish the prolactin response to suckling in the first week postpartum, *Pediatrics*, 113: 465–571.

RCPCH UK-WHO (2013) *UK-WHO Growth Charts-0–4 Years*. Available online at www.rcpch.ac.uk/resources/uk-who-growth-charts-0-4-years (accessed 1 May 2022)

Regan, S. and Brown, A. (2019) Experiences of online breastfeeding support: Support and reassurance versus judgement and misinformation, *Maternal & Child Nutrition*, 15: e12874. Available online at https://doi.org/10.1111/mcn.12874 (accessed 1 January 2023)

Renfrew, M., Ansell, P. and MacLeod, K. (2003) Formula feed preparation – helping reduce the risks: A systematic review, Archives of Disease in Childhood, 88(10): 855–858

Renfrew, M., Dyson, L., McCormick, E., *et al.* (2009) Breastfeeding promotion for infants in neonatal units: A systematic review, Child: Care, Health and Development, 36(2): 165–178

Renfrew, M., Dyson, L., Wallace, L., *et al.* (2005) The Effectiveness of Public Health Interventions to Promote the Duration of Breastfeeding: Systematic Review, London: NICE

Renfrew, M., McLoughlin, M. and McFadden, A. (2008) Cleaning and sterilisation of infant feeding equipment: A systematic review, Public Health Nutrition, 11(11): 1188–1199

Renfrew, M., Pokhrel, S., Quigley, M., *et al.* (2012) Preventing Disease and Saving Resources: The Potential Contribution of Increasing Breastfeeding Rates in the UK, London: UNICEF UK. Available online at The Baby Friendly Initiative | Resources | Preventing disease and saving resources (unicef.org.uk) (accessed 1 October 2022)

Renfrew, M., Woolridge, M. and McGill, H. (2000) Enabling Women to Breastfeed: A Review of Practices Which Promote or Inhibit Breastfeeding – With Evidence-Based Guidance for Practice, London: The Stationery Office

Riddle, S. and Nommsen-Rivers, L. (2016) A case control study of diabetes during pregnancy and low milk supply, *Breastfeed Med*, 11(2): 80–85

Roller, C. (2005) Getting to know mothers' experiences of kangaroo care, *Journal of Obstetrics, Gynaecology and Neonatal Nursing*, 34: 210–217

Rollins, N., Bhandari, N., Hajeebhoy, N., *et al.* (2016) Why invest and what will it take to improve breastfeeding practices? *The Lancet*, 387(10017), 491–504

Rollins, N., Piwoz, E., Baker., P., *et al.* (2023) Marketing of commercial milk formula: A system to capture parents, communities, science, and policy, *The Lancet*, 401(10375): 486–502

Rollnick, S., Miller, W. and Butler, C. (2008) Motivational Interviewing in Healthcare; Helping Patients Change Behaviour, New York: The Guildford Press

Rosenthal, P. (2014) Another explanation for breast milk jaundice, The Journal of Pediatrics, 165(1): 10–11

Royal College of Midwives (RCM) (2009) Infant Feeding: A Resource for Health Care Professionals and Parents, London: RCM Trust

Royal College of Midwives (RCM) (2020) Parental Emotional Wellbeing and Infant Development, London: RCM

Royal College of Obstetricians and Gynaecologist (RCOG) (2018) *Care of Women with Obesity in Pregnancy (Green Top Guideline No. 72)*. Available online at www.rcog.org.uk (accessed 19 January 2023)

Royal College of Obstetricians and Gynaecologist (RCOG) (2022) *Coronavirus (Covid-19), Infection and Pregnancy FAQs*. Available online at www.rcog.org.uk (accessed 14 January 2023)

Rozga, M., Kerver, J. and Olson, B. (2014) Self-reported reasons for breastfeeding cessation among low income women enrolled in a peer counselling breastfeeding support program, *Journal of Human Lactation*, *31*(1). Available online at https://doi-org.knowledge.idm.oclc.org/10.1177/0890334414548070 (accessed 12 January 2023)

Sackett, D., Rosenberg, W., Gray, J., *etal.* (1996) Evidence based medicine: What it is and what it isn't, *British Medical Journal*, 312: 71–72

Schaal, B., Doucet, S., Sagot, P., *et al.* (2005) Human breast areolae as scent organs: Morphological data and possible involvement in maternal – neonatal condition, *Developmental Psychobiology*, 48: 100–110

Schiff, M., Algert, C., Ampt, A., *et al.* (2014) The impact of cosmetic breast implants on breastfeeding: A systematic review and meta-analysis, *International Breastfeeding Journal*, 9: 17. Available online at www.ncbi.nlm.nih.gov/pmc/articles/PMC4203468 (accessed 19 January 2023)

Schön, D. (1983) The Reflective Practitioner, New York: Basic Books

Schore, A. (2001) dysregulation of the right brain: A fundamental mechanism of traumatic attachment and the psychopathogenesis of posttraumatic stress disorder, *Australian and New Zealand Journal of Psychiatry*, 36: 9–30

Scientific Advisory Committee on Nutrition (SACN) (2008) *Consideration of the Place of 'Good Night' Milk Products in the Diet of Infants Aged 6 Months*. Available online at www.gov.uk/government/publications/sacn-statement-on-good-night-milks-2008(accessed 22 January 2023)

Scientific Advisory Committee on Nutrition (SACN) (2016) *Vitamin D and Health*. Available online at www.gov.uk/government/publications/sacn-vitamin-d-and-health-report (accessed 12 October 2022)

Scientific Advisory Committee on Nutrition (SACN) (2018) *Feeding in the First Year of Life*. Available online at https://ww w.gov.uk/government/publications/sacn-report-on-feeding-in-the-first-year-of-life (accessed 14 August 2022)

Scottish Government (SG) (2017) *Scottish Maternal and Infant Nutrition Survey*. Available online at www.gov.scot (accessed 05 August 2022)

Scottish Government (SG) (2021) *Trauma-Informed Practice: A Toolkit for Scotland*. Available online at www.gov.scot/publications/trauma-informed-practice-toolkit-scotland/ (accessed 24 January 2023)

Shaker, C. (2013) Cue-based co-regulated feeding in the neonatal intensive care unit: Supporting parents in learning to feed their preterm infant. Newborn and Infant Nursing Reviews, 13(1): 51–55

Sheriff, N., Hall, V. and Pickin, M. (2009) Fathers' perspectives on breastfeeding: Ideas for intervention, British Journal of Midwifery, 17(4): 223–227

Sheriff, N., Panton, C. and Hall, V. (2014) A new model of father support to promote breastfeeding, Community Practitioner, 87(5): 20–24

Sihota, H., Oliffes, J., Jelly, M., *et al.* (2019) Father's experiences and perspectives of breastfeeding: A scoping review, *American Journal of Men's Health*, 13(3): 1–12

Silvers, K., Frampton, C., Wickens, K., *et al.* (2012) breastfeeding protects against current asthma up to 6 years of age, The Journal of Pediatrics, 160(6): 991–996

Simmer, K., Patole, S. and Rao, S. (2017) Longchain polyunsaturated fatty acid supplementation in infants born at term, *Cochrane Database of Systematic Reviews*. Available online at https://doi.org/10.1002/14651858.CD000376.pub4 (accessed 22 January 2023)

Sinkiewicz-Darol, E., Bernatowicz- Lojko, U., Lubiech, K., *et al.* (2021) Tandem breastfeeding: A descriptive analysis of the nutritional value of milk when feeding a younger and older child, *Nutrients, 13*(1): 277

Specialist Pharmacy Service (SPS) (2020) *Safety in Lactation: Viral Hepatitis*, Specialist Pharmacy Service, NHS. Available online at www.sps.nhs.uk (accessed 13 January 2023)

Spencer, J. (2008) Management of mastitis in breastfeeding women, American Family Physician, 78(6): 727–833

Stenhouse, E. (2018) Breastfeeding and diabetes, in D. McCance, M. Maresh and D. Sacks (eds) *A Practical Manual of Diabetes in Pregnancy* (2nd edn), Chichester: John Wiley & Sons

Stevens, J., Schmied, V., Burns, E. and Dahlen, H. (2014) Immediate or early skin-to-skin contact after a caesarean section: A review of the literature, *Maternal and Child Nutrition*, 10: 456–473

Stiles, J. and Jernigan, T. (2010) The basics of brain development, *Neuropsychology Review*, 20(4): 327–348. Available online at www.ncbi.nlm.nih.gov/pmc/articles/PMC2989000/ (accessed 27 October 2022)

Svensson, K., Velandia, M., Matthiesen, A., *et al.* (2013) Effects of mother-infant skin-to-skin contact on severe latch-on problems in older infants: A randomized trial. *International Breastfeeding Journal*, 8: 1. Available online at https://internationalbreastfeedingjournal.biomedcentral.com/articles/10.1186/1746-4358-8-1#citeas (accessed 6 January 2023)

Taylor, C., Tully, K. and Ball, H. (2015) Night-time on a postnatal ward: Experiences of mothers, infants, and staff, in *Ethnographic Research in Maternal and Child Health*, Abingdon, Oxon: Routledge, 117–140

Teplica, D., Cooney, E., Jeffers, E., *et al.* (2022) There is no 'Axillary Tail': Rethinking the assumption of James Spence, *Plastic Reconstruction Surgery Global Open*, 10(2): e4086. Available online at www.ncbi.nlm.nih.gov/pmc/articles/PMC8830835/ (accessed 6 January 2023)

Thompson, J., Heal, L., Roberts, C., *et al.* (2010) Women's breastfeeding experiences following a significant primary postpartum haemorrhage: A multicentre cohort study, *International Breastfeeding Journal*. Available online at https://internationalbreastfeedingjournal.biomedcentral.com/articles/10.1186/1746-4358-5-5(accessed 18 January 2023)

Thomson, G. and Crossland, N. (2019) Using the behaviour change wheel to explore infant feeding peer support provision; insights from a North West UK evaluation, *International Breastfeeding Journal*, 14(41). Available online at https://internationalbreastfeedingjournal.biomedcentral.com/articles/10.1186/s13006-019-0236-7 (accessed 4 January 2023)

Toscano, M., De Grandi, R., Peroni, D., *et al.* (2017) Impact of delivery mode on the colostrum microbiota composition, *BMC Microbiology*. Available online at https://bmcmicrobiol.biomedcentral.com/articles/10.1186/s12866-017-1109-0 (accessed 12 October 2022)

Trimeloni, L. and Spencer, J. (2016) Diagnosis and management of breast milk oversupply, Journal of the American Board of Family Medicine, 29(1): 139–242

Trotter, S. (2010) Raising awareness amongst parents of treatments for tongue-tie, MIDIRS Midwifery Digest, 20(1): 83–85

Turcksin, R., Bel, S., Galjaard, S., *et al.* (2013) Maternal obesity and breastfeeding intention, initiation, intensity and duration: A systematic review, Maternal and Child Nutrition, 10(2): 1–18.

UNICEF UK BFI (2002) *Introducing the Baby Friendly Best Practice Standards into Breastfeeding Education for Student Midwives and Health Visitors*, London: UNICEF UK Baby Friendly Initiative

UNICEF UK BFI (2014) *A Guide to Infant Formula for Parents Who Are Bottle Feeding: The Health Professionals'.* Available online at www.unicef.org.uk/babyfriendly/wp-content/uploads/sites/2/2016/12/Health-professionals-guide-to-infant-formula.pdf (accessed 15th August 2022)

UNICEF UK BFI (2016a) *Protecting Health and Saving Lives: A Call to Action*, Chap 1. Available online at www.unicef.org.uk/babyfriendly (accessed 9 October 2022)

UNICEF UK BFI (2016b) *Responsive Feeding: Supporting Close and Loving Relationships*. Available online at www.unicef.org.uk/babyfriendly (accessed 18 October 2022)

UNICEF UK BFI (2017a) *Guide to the UNICEF UK Baby Friendly Initiative Standards*. Available online at www.unicef.org.uk/babyfriendly (accessed 30 April 2022)

UNICEF UK BFI (2017b) *Assessment of Breastmilk Expression*. Available online at www.unicef.org.uk/babyfriendly (accessed 18 October 2022)

UNICEF UK BFI (2019a) *Guide to the UNICEF UK Baby Friendly Initiative University Standards*. Available online at www.unicef.org.uk/babyfriendly (accessed 30 April 2022)

UNICEF UK BFI (2019b) *Responsive Bottle Feeding*. Available online at www.unicef.org.uk/babyfriendly (accessed 18 October 2022)

UNICEF UK BFI (2021) Building a Happy Baby. A Guide for Parents, London: UNICEF UK

UNICEF UK BFI (2022) Guide to the UNICEF UK Baby Friendly Initiative Neonatal Standards for Neonatal Units, London: UNICEF UK

UNICEF UK BFI (n.d.) *Guidance for Antenatal and Postnatal Conversations*. London: UNICEF UK. Available online at www.unicef.org.uk/babyfriendly/baby-friendly-resources/implementing-standards-resources/guidance-for-antenatal-and-postnatal-conversations/ (accessed 12 December 2022)

Uvnäs-Moberg, K., Ekström-Bergstöm, A., Buckley, S., *et al.* (2020) Maternal plasma levels of oxytocin during breastfeeding: A systematic review, *PLoS ONE*, 15(8): e0235806. Available online at https://doi.org/10.1371/journal.pone.0235806 (accessed 17 October 2022)

Van der Wijden, C. and Manion, C. (2015) Lactational amenorrhoea method for family planning, *Cochrane Database of Systematic Reviews*. Available online at https://doi.org/10.1002%2F1465 1858.CD001329.pub2 (accessed 4 January 2023)

van Veldhuizen-Staas, C. (2007) Overabundant milk supply: An alternative way to intervene by full drainage and block feeding, *International Breastfeeding Journal*, 2(11). Available online at www.ncbi.nlm.nih.gov/pmc/articles/PMC2075483 (accessed 6 January 2023)

Verret-Chalifour, J., Giguère, Y., Forest, J.C., *et al.* (2015) Breastfeeding initiation: Impact of obesity in a large Canadian perinatal cohort study, *PLoS ONE*, 10(2): e0117512

Victora, C., Bahl, R., Barros, A., *et al.* (2016) Breastfeeding in the 21st century: Epidemiology, mechanisms, and lifelong effect, *The Lancet*, 387(10017): 475–490

Wambach, K. and Riordan, J. (2016) Breastfeeding and Human Lactation, Burlington, MA: Jones and Bartlett Publishers

Wang, S., Guendelman, S., Harley, K., *et al.* (2018) When fathers are perceived to share in the maternal decision to breastfeed: Outcomes from the infant feeding practices survey II, *Maternal & Child Health Journal*, 22: 1676–1684

Watson, J. and McGuire, W. (2016) Responsive versus scheduled feeding for pre-term infants, *Cochrane Database of Systematic Reviews*. Available online at https://doi.org/10.1002/14651858.CD005255.pub5 (accessed 5 January 2023)

Watson-Genna, C. and Rabin, J. (2022) Breastfeeding: Normal sucking and swallowing, in C. Watson-Genna (eds) Supporting Sucking Skills in Breastfeeding Infants (4th edn), Burlington, MA: Jones and Bartlett Publishers.

White, J. (1995) Patterns of knowing: Review, critique, and update, Advances in Nursing Science, 17(4): 73–86

Widström, A., Lija, G., Aaltomaa-Michalias, P., *et al.* (2011) Newborn behaviour to locate the breast when skin-to-skin: A possible method for enabling early self-regulation, *Acta Paediatrica*, 100(1): 79–85

Wilde, C., Addey, C., Boddy, L., *et al.* (1995) Autocrine regulation of milk secretion by a protein in milk, Biochemistry Journal, 1(305): 51–58

Wilson, C., Finch, E., Kerr, C., et al. (2020) Alcohol, smoking and other substance use in the perinatal period, *British Medical Journal*, 369: 1627. Available online at https://doi.org/10.1136/bmj.m1627 (accessed 15 January 2023)

World Alliance for Breastfeeding Action (WABA) (2005) *Towards Healthy Environments for Children: FAQs about Breastfeeding in a Contaminated Environment*. Available online at www.waba.org.my/whatwedo/environment/pdf/faq2005_eng.pdf (accessed 27 October 2022)

World Health Organization (WHO) (1981) International Code of Marketing of Breast Milk Substitutes, Geneva: WHO

World Health Organization (WHO) (1990) Innocenti Declaration on the Protection, Promotion and Support of Breastfeeding, Florence: WHO

World Health Organization (WHO) (1998a) Evidence for the Ten Steps to Successful Breastfeeding, Geneva: WHO

World Health Organization (WHO) (1998b) Relactation: Review of Experience and Recommendations for Practice, Geneva: WHO

World Health Organization (WHO) (2010) Guidelines on HIV and Infant Feeding: Principles and Recommendations for Infant Feeding in the Context of HIV and a Summary of Evidence, Geneva: WHO.

World Health Organization (WHO) (2014a) *Global Nutrition Targets 2025. Breastfeeding Policy Brief 5*. Available online at www.who.int/publications/i/item/WHO-NMH-NHD-14.7 (accessed 28 October 2022)

World Health Organization (WHO) (2014b) Guideline for the Identification and Management of Substance Use and Substance Use Disorders in Pregnancy, Geneva: WHO

World Health Organization (WHO) (2016) Guideline Updates on HIV and Breastfeeding. The Duration of Breastfeeding and Support from Health Services to Improve Feeding Practices Among Mothers Living with HIV, Geneva: WHO

World Health Organization (WHO) (2018) Ten Steps to Successful Breastfeeding. Available online at www.who.int/teams/nutrition-and-food-safety/food-and-nutrition-actions-in-health-systems/ten-steps-to-successful-breastfeeding (accessed 25 January 2023)

World Health Organization (WHO) (2020) *Breastfeeding and Covid-19: Scientific Brief*, Geneva: WHO

World Health Organization (WHO) (2021a) *Infant and Young Child Feeding*, Geneva: WHO Available online at Infant and young child feeding (who.int) (accessed 18 October 2022)

World Health Organization (WHO) (2021b) *Immediate 'Kangaroo Mother Care' and Survival of Infants with Low Birth Wight*, Geneva: WHO. Available online at www.who.int/news/item/26-05-2021-kangaroo-mother-care-started-immediately-after-birth-critical-for-saving-lives-new-research-shows (accessed 5 January 2023)

World Health Organization (WHO) (2023) *Nutrition, Breastfeeding*. Available online at https://apps.who.int/nutrition/topics/exclusive_breastfeeding/en/ (accessed 4 January 2023)

World Health Organization (WHO)/UNICEF (1989) Ten Steps to Successful Breastfeeding, Geneva: WHO. Available online at Nutrition and Food Safety (who.int) (accessed 27 October 2022)

World Health Organization (WHO)/UNICEF (2009) Acceptable Medical Reasons for the Use of Breast-Milk Substitutes, Geneva: WHO

World Health Organization (WHO)/UNICEF (2021) *Global Breastfeeding Scorecard 2021*. Available online at https://apps.who.int/iris/bitstream/handle/10665/348546/WHO-HEP-NFS-21.45-eng.pdf?sequence=1 (accessed 4 January 2023)

Yan, J., Liu, L., Zhu, Y., *et al.* (2014) The Association between breastfeeding and childhood obesity: A meta-analysis, BMC Public Health, 14(1): 1267

Young, C., Kingma, S. and Neu, J. (2011) Ischemia-reperfusion and neonatal intestinal injury, The Journal of Pediatrics, 158(2): 25–28

Zakarija-Grkovic, I. and Stewart, F. (2020) Treatments for breast engorgement, *Cochrane Database of Systematic Reviews*. Available online at https://doi.org/10.1002/14651858.CD006946.pub4 (accessed 12 January 2023)

Zimmerman, E. and Thompson, K. (2015) Clarifying nipple confusion, *Journal of Perinatology*, 35: 895–899

Index

Note: numbers in **bold** indicate a table

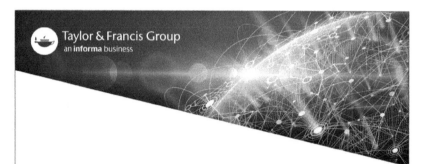

Printed in the USA
CPSIA information can be obtained
at www.ICGtesting.com
LVHW060553170924
791293LV00007B/735

9 781032 252407